An Easy Guide On How to Establish Your First Residential Care Facility

Small Family Home, SFH
Foster Family Home, FFH
Foster Family Agency, FFA
Group Home, GH
Transitional Housing, THPF
Adult Residential Care Facility, ARF
Residential Care Facility for the Elderly, RCFE
Residential Care Facility for the Chronically Ill, RFCI

By
Romwell Martinez Sabeniano, MBA. HCM

authorHOUSE™

1663 LIBERTY DRIVE, SUITE 200
BLOOMINGTON, INDIANA 47403
(800) 839-8640
WWW.AUTHORHOUSE.COM

© 2005 Romwell Martinez Sabeniano, MBA.HCM. All Rights Reserved.

No part of this book may be reproduced, stored in a retrieval system, or transmitted by any means without the written permission of the author.

First published by AuthorHouse 03/24/05

ISBN: 1-4208-3357-X (sc)
ISBN: 1-4208-4475-X (e)

Library of Congress Control Number: 2005901299

Printed in the United States of America
Bloomington, Indiana

This book is printed on acid-free paper.

The information presented in this book is readily accessible from public agencies and offices and is deemed reliable at the time of printing. It is recommended that the reader should seek advice and consultation from other health care professionals, consultants, legal counsels and other entities relative to their particular undertaking. The author is not rendering professional advice but rather presenting useful materials for beginners in the business. Individual results may vary and the author does not guarantee the success of each and everyone's undertaking. State and Federal regulations may change from time to time, as agency rules, procedures and budgetary considerations could affect the future results of the business. The information stated herein are acquired from existing regulations, general principles, guidelines and practices observed in a typical residential care and institutional setting and are deemed in effect at the time this book was printed. It is the responsibility of the reader to keep abreast of the latest changes in regulations and guidelines that could affect their respective residential care business. This book is sold and is purchased by the reader with the understanding that the author and its publisher are not engaged in rendering legal or professional service. Notwithstanding anything to the contrary stated or implied in any of the materials available herein, the author as well as Health Care Training and Staffing Services, its agents, affiliates, employees and contractors cannot and do not make any representation, warranty, endorsement or guarantee, express or implied, regarding (i) the accuracy, completeness or timeliness of any such information, facts or opinions or (ii) the merchantability or fitness for any particular purpose thereof, nor shall any of such materials be deemed the giving of legal advice by the author, Health Care Training and Staffing Services, its agents, affiliates, employees or contractors.

Acknowledgments

This book is a compilation of the knowledge and the resources that I accumulated from more than 12 years of experience in the health care field. Through the years of my lifetime, there is a lot of things I am very grateful for and owe my sincerest thanks to the people I love and care about. First and foremost I thank GOD for all the blessings and the challenges HE has given me and my family. To my devoted and loving wife Cecilia who is always there for me and I truly love her dearly, and to my charming and intelligent daughter Ysabel who is my love and inspiration, to my son Miguel Antonio who with his brief stay with us he shared lasting memories we will never forget. To my dearest mother Modesta Rosario Sabeniano, my dad Ernesto V. Martinez and my father and mother–in-law Juan and Sonia Vasconcellos, my sisters Myriam, Judith, Carol and my brother JoyDennis. Special thanks to my brothers and sisters in-law Jose and Lillian, Niles, Marion, Peter, John, Robert and Carrie, for their love and unwavering support, to my nephews and nieces Ciarra, Ennio, Hamilton, Carolina, David, Nathan, Seth and to all the "special people" I meet on a daily basis who have touched my life and as a result, became my friends. I am also grateful to Etta May Cable, Rey G., Susan K, and to those who are disabled, the abused, the neglected and the elderly whom I established a bonding friendship through all these years; to all my staff, my publisher, to Ms. Marylyn Hope who helped in editing my book, and to those who contributed in any way by making this book finally complete after four years of concentrated effort. And lastly, I want to thank all the dreamers, the believers, the visionaries, and the readers of this book. I thank you all sincerely from the bottom of my heart.

Romwell Martinez Sabeniano, MBA.HCM
Author-Publisher

Table of Contents

Acknowledgments vii

INTRODUCTION xxvii

Chapter 1: UNDERSTANDING THE RESIDENTIAL CARE BUSINESS 1

THE FACILITY: A Perspective. 1
    I.   Learning the Business. 1
    II. What is long-term care? 5
    III. Who needs long-term care? 5
    IV. What are the different types of long-term care services available? 6
SMALL FAMILY HOME (SFH) 11
FOSTER FAMILY HOME (FFH) 12
FOSTER FAMILY AGENCY (FFA) 12
TRANSITIONAL HOUSING (TH) 12
GROUP HOME (GH) 13
ADULT RESIDENTIAL FACILITY (ARF) 14
RESIDENTIAL CARE FACILITY FOR THE ELDERLY (RCFE) 14
RESIDENTIAL CARE FACILITY FOR THE CHRONICALLY ILL (RCFCI) 14
ADULT DAY CARE FACILITY (ADCF) / SOCIAL DAY CARE (SDCF) 14
TRANSITIONAL HOUSING 14
    V.   What standards apply to long-term care facilities? 23
    VI. What is the role of the state in the welfare system? 23
    VII. FACTS ABOUT LONG-TERM CARE 25

Chapter 2: GETTING STARTED IN THE BUSINESS 27

Create a Checklist 27

"HOW TO" STEPS IN SETTING UP THE COMMUNITY CARE
FACILITY BUSINESS... 28
- B. Things to consider when establishing the facility:................ 34
- C. Checklist of important things to remember in keeping the facility operation within the required licensing standards. ... 35
- D. Types of Consumers/Clients Placed in Residential Care Facilities 41
- E. Levels of care is equivalent to the level of pay for the services provided. 43
- F. How do you get paid for the services provided in the facility and who pays for the long-term care services?..................... 54

Chapter 3: THE ORIENTATION 65

- A. THE THREE COMPONENTS OF THE APPLICATION PROCESS.. 66
- B. WHAT ARE THE DIFFERENT FORMS NEEDED TO COMPLETE THE APPLICATION 67

Chapter 4: THE FACILITY ADMINISTRATOR CERTIFICATION COURSE.. 91

Step 2. BECOME A CERTIFIED FACILITY ADMINISTRATOR... 91

Chapter 5: THE BUSINESS PLAN 105

Step 3. Create a Business Plan 105
A Business Plan 105
- A. THE START UP COST 107
  SAMPLE START UP COST 108

Chapter 6: FINANCING THE BUSINESS.................................... 111

- A. FREE MONEY: WHERE TO SECURE FINANCING, FREE MONEY, GRANTS, GIFTS DONATIONS, ETC... TO FINANCE THE BUSINESS... 111
- 1. Personal funds, money from friends and relatives, get a business partner, look for an investor: 112

2. Regional Centers, Probation, Dept. of Aging and other Placement Agencies: 113
3. US Small Business Administration (SBA). 113
4. Fannie Mae: 115
5. US Department of Housing and Urban Development (HUD): US Dept. of HUD, has various programs that the reader might want to explore. 115
    (a). Title 1 Housing and Community Development Act of 1974 115
    (b). Community Development Block Grants: 115
    (c). HOPE for Homeownership of Single Family Homes: .. 116
    (d). Shelter Plus (S+C): 116
    (e). Supportive Housing for Persons with Disabilities:......... 116
    (f). Department of Housing & Community Development:..... 116
    (g). PRIVATE PHILATHROPIC FOUNDATIONS: 117

WRITING A GRANT PROPOSAL 117
Components of a Proposal/ GRANT 118
BUY A HOUSE WITH LITTLE DOWN OR USING CREATIVE FINANCING? 119

Chapter 7: PROGRAM DESIGN 121

Step 4: Prepare a Draft of the Program Design................................ 121
WHAT IS A PROGRAM DESIGN ? 124
Contents of a Program Design 125
PROCESS FOR SUBMISSION OF INITIAL PROGRAM STATEMENT 126

Chapter 8: THE BUSINESS ENTITY 131

Step 5: Establish your Business Entity 131
Sole Proprietorship, Corporation (For profit or Non- Profit), Partnership, Limited Liability Corporation.............................. 131
What is an Article of Incorporation? 135
What is the Board of Directors? 137
FICTITIOUS BUSINESS NAME 149

File for Fictitious Business Name Statement 149
BUSINESS LICENSE 150

Chapter 9: ACQUIRE THE PROPERTY/BUSINESS 153

What type of house is allowed in residential care setting, residential or commercial? 154
What and where is a good location to put up a residential care facility? 154
Step 6:   Acquire the Business/Real Estate property on lease or purchase 155
The 300 Feet Rule: 160
LEASE WITH OPTION TO PURCHASE: 160
Things to consider when buying a property for the business 162
SALE-LEASE BACK 163

Chapter 10: THE HOST LETTER 165

Step 7:   Secure Host Letter 165

Chapter 11: INSURANCE COVERAGE 167

Step 8:   Get your facility insured 167

Chapter 12: SUBMITTING THE APPLICATION PACKET ... 169

Step 9:   Submit the Application for a License to Operate a Facility. (Second Stage/Component) 169
Step 10: Request for Fire Marshal to Inspect the Facility and Request for Certification 171

Chapter 13: RESPONDING TO A REQUEST FOR PROPOSAL (RFP) 175

Q&A on Request for a Proposal 175

Chapter 14: VENDORIZATION 179

Step 11. Secure Vendorization Packet: 179
What is Regional Center? 180

Step 12: Community Care Licensing Representative to visit the facility to confirm compliance with the regulation (Third Stage / Component). 187
Step 13: Approval of License to Operate. Issuance of Provisional License (if no pending major issues on the application). 188
Step 14: Business Officially Begins upon receipt of a provisional license to operate. 189

EXHIBIT ONE: SAMPLE ARTICLES OF INCORPORATION AND BY-LAWS **190**

EXHIBIT TWO: SAMPLE PROGRAM DESIGN **229**

EXHIBIT THREE: : SAMPLE BUSINESS PLAN **329**

Why is this book important to you in setting up your caregiving business?

This book was written especially for those who are considering the idea of getting into the business of providing a service in a residential care setting particularly those who are exploring this business potential for the first time but have little or no experience at all. It is also for those who have a lot of courage and determination to succeed, but may have very limited money to start up the business, this book is for you. Contrary to what other people think, anyone can succeed and make a lot of money in this business.

This book is also for those who need help in starting a residential care business and keeping it going. It is also to help those who are interested in establishing their first residential care business despite their limitations and challenges in setting up the business not knowing what to do and where to start. It also serves as an easy guide to the inexperienced self-starters who could use some helpful hints when going through the whole process from start to finish. It eliminates all the confusion that beginners in the business normally encounter particularly to those who do not have any idea on what to do first, who to turn to next, what agency to approach and when, where to look for the best location for their facility, what form to fill out, how to get funding, etc...

Are we going to be rich in the business? Perhaps, that answer depends on the individual's perspective. In my experience, there are people I met in the business who persevered long enough to be able to afford to live in lavishly designed million dollar homes and drive fancy cars, wear designer clothes and maintain an incredible lifestyle of financial freedom, able to take extended vacation to exotic places and countries any time they desire.

There are also those who have gotten tired working in the business for so many years and decided that a job in their own business is no longer their idea of retirement, so they sold the property and its potential income in exchange for a comfortable lifestyle free from stress and anxiety. However, do not get me wrong. There are also quite a number of people who are no longer in the businesses and lost their homes for one reason or another, some figured out that the business was not for them because of the loss of hundreds or thousands of hard-earned dollars in the business.

Is the business going to work well for us? For those among us who are looking for a business that will make them rich overnight, to be honest, this is not that kind of business. It will take a lot of patience, dedication and hard work. If we are willing to nurture it and watch it grow as we genuinely provide the best care that we can offer, in time, yes we will be compensated accordingly depending on the effort that we exert. What is important now is for us to do our best in serving others, and money will come in unexpected amount and from various places as long as we manage the business well.

Most, if not all, have the goal of achieving the great American dream of establishing a business, and being free from working as an employee for the rest of their life. However, some might just be contented with working from one job to another to supplement their income. Others enjoy the idea of going home from work everyday then going back to work the next day for the next 15 to 20 years. Quite a number will decide to work for someone else and help make that person get wealthy instead. The sad part of it is when we do not know other options but to work hard for as long as we can. There is nothing wrong with that. What really matters is we enjoy what it is that we do with our life. But, the question remains… as we age every second of our lifetime, we will realize that there are things we used to do, that for reasons other than physical, financial or medical reasons, we can no longer do them today. How long can we keep doing what we are doing right now? Unless we embrace the winds of change, we will remain stuck where we are and for whatever it is. Are we willing to keep doing that which we have been doing for the next 10 to 30 years? Are we going to look for another part time second or third job, are we waiting for someone else like our boss to decide for us until that one day when we can no longer keep our jobs because the company closed its business or has outsourced the jobs to another country where cost of labor is cheaper? It is indeed alarming to know that in reality, such is the fact in our daily life that we need to face now or someday we will have to. I do not know about your plans, but to me I will not sit down and wait to rely upon someone else to decide on what my destiny will bring. Honestly speaking, I know that deep inside you, there is the burning desire to create a positive result out of your current financial situation whatever it is. We all have the power to decide for ourselves what our future may bring. Otherwise, you would not have bought this book nor attended the required orientation on the subject of residential care business, right? What orientation do I mean? If you are reading this book right now and have not attended the initial orientation course required by your local Community Care Licensing Agency or the Health Care Licensing organization, do not panic. You are still on the right track. I will discuss this topic later on in this book.

Most if not everyone wants to take control of their destiny by establishing an enterprise they call their own and be the "BOSS". We hope that some day the business we aim to establish will grow until it becomes our big break in getting out of our current situation, whatever it is whether it be unemployment, to get rid of our unwanted jobs and do something while on retirement, or we have a property that we want to generate income potentials from.

No matter what reason that drives us to set up this business, it is important that we understand our goal and the mission that we are trying to accomplish. We need to have something that will drive our determination to make the business work no matter what it takes. There must be some form of a reality check for us to make an honest evaluation of ourselves what is it that we want to accomplish and if we have decided yet on our plan to succeed in this business. No matter how grandiose or small our dream business may be, whether it be a "board and care home" business or a store that will sell widgets, there is one thing we will surely find out later.... any dream business will take a lot of hard work, patience and sacrifices in order to may even possibly come true. Even if we try our best in getting the business together, even if we have all the resources and the talent that qualify us to become successful in the business, still there are no guarantees that the business we have in mind will succeed or even make it to the first year. Studies show that 95% of start-up businesses fail during the first three years of operation. Even then, a big portion of those who succeed on the first year might not even make it by the fifth year in operation. It is quite alarming but, if we do not try at all, we will never find out what is possible for ourselves.

There are a lot of things we need to know initially about the residential care business if that is what we want to do. There is a substantial amount of information to absorb before we should plunge into the business with our hard-earned money. Not having any idea at all on what to do and how to go about it may be a very frightening thought, especially to those of us who have limited cash and minimal experience.

Realistically, at this stage, the hardest thing to do is deciding when to start. Later on in the process, you will realize when you look back from this challenging new experience that was indeed worth a try as you will have learned a lot of things from it and found out that it was not as hard as you thought it was.

Let me make it clear however, that this book will not serve as the only solution to all the questions about the business as individual situation or experiences may vary. However, with the selective information presented in this book, you will feel confident on what you need to do in the process. It will serve as a map to plot your directions and assure you that you no longer feel lost in the dark not knowing what to expect in this business.

In life, do not allow yourself to be overwhelmed by the environment, by the negative things around you and most of all not to fall into the trap of being unprepared for what you are about to face in your new business.

By purchasing this book, you have practically made that BIG DECISION to start and get the wheels in motion, which is a good sign. What is important now is for you to read and absorb the available information in this book, analyze your current situation and try to picture where you want to be when you accomplish your objective. You will need to evaluate your finances, make a plan on how you are going to accomplish it and most of all solidify your commitment to make your dream business a reality.

As you embark for the first time in accepting the different challenges in your new business, you will realize how important your role is as a provider of care. In due time, you will experience a unique kind of feeling that no one can describe unless they themselves have experienced what you are about to experience caring for others. Eventually, you will become part of other people's lives as they consider you as an advocate, a friend or an ally particularly to the aged and for individuals who are physically, mentally or developmentally challenged. Your role should you decide to accept it, is indeed very important. You are about to take care of the need of the future today not only in this population or environment but you are also contributing to the global solution on caring.

Is there a demand for the business? YES, DEFINITELY. The type of facility and its location partly determines how busy you will be with your business. Every successful business requires the right location. You must choose a location in an area where there is no over supply of the same category/type of facility or service. Remember, you are not just in the business of serving the needs of the community but you are also in real estate business. You will eventually realize that no matter what the global economy brings, there will always be a need for your business. Look around you seriously. There is an estimated 87 million Americans most of whom belong to the "Baby Boomers" generation. These include those who will turn 65 years old between 1990 and year 2020. The fact of the matter is that, eventually, we will all age. As we do, we will all have to make that decision to prepare ourselves for the inevitable aging process by accepting our age at our private homes and have someone take care of us or to by living with a group of people in a facility/residential care setting. Every day we face that uncertainty in our health where we are challenged by the possibilities of developing some form of unexpected disability beyond our control such as diseases, accident or by some genetic fluke where all of a sudden we are confronted by medical challenges that could make us bedfast for a long time. It may sound like a scary line from a horror movie but it is the truth. There are approximately 50 million Americans with disability and in the San Bernardino and Riverside Counties alone, there are more than 20,000 people with some form of developmental disability who need help.

Your business will be able to accommodate only a fraction of that aging and disabled population but undoubtedly, there is the need for your services no matter what our respective state budget dictates on a yearly basis.

If you were to ask, "How long will it take to set the business up and running?" I would guesstimate that you would be able to get it started from scratch to full operation within at least six to eight months or less depending on how soon you can meet all the requirements, how efficient you are in helping your respective local community care agency, your designated licensing program analyst in evaluating your program design, where the home will be located and the demand as well as the availability of resources in the area where your business will be established and whole lot of things that will be discussed later on in this book as you go along with your reading.

YOU NEED THIS BOOK TO GET STARTED WITH EASE

- *Your road map to building your residential care facility.* This book will help you go through the process of building the business and to possibly limit the anxiety of making a guess work effort on your part thereby reducing the frequencies of your error. Instead of making a ton of mistakes wandering around what needs to be done or if you miss anything significant that could affect the outcome of your effort, this book will certainly serve as a guide map towards the direction of setting up the business right from the beginning.

- *Save your frustrations and get some relief.* This book will give you relief from the anxiety of not knowing where to start and how to get it going. Its role is very important in helping your understanding of what it takes to get the business up and running, what to expect from the business and what the business expects from you in return. The book will also help you set your goals and expectation in the business, to give you a better picture of how you are doing in the process, to help you understand how the whole process works and formulate some ideas on what steps to take to enable yourself to complete the process from start to finish.

- *Save yourself thousands of dollars in consultation fees*. With this book is included **FREE SAMPLE PROGRAM DESIGNS, FREE SAMPLE BUSINESS OPERATIONS FORMS, SAMPLE BY-LAWS, ETC...** that you can use as an example guide when you draw your own program design. In order to be a licensed facility, one of the requirements is to write your own program design describing the facility in writing, its operations and procedures, its roles and responsibilities and lot of things to describe the facility that you want to establish. That same program design that you draw up will be similar to what you will need to prepare when you meet with your local vendorizing agency such as Regional Center, Dept. of Probation, Dept. of Aging etc... You will find out later on in the early stages of this undertaking that drawing your own program design without any serious professional help or the basic knowledge of the Title 22 and Title 17 Regulation would make your initial application stage extremely difficult. People find out after attending the initial orientation from

Community Care Licensing that just the task of drawing their own program design alone is enough reason for them to quit at the beginning because it does take a considerable amount of perseverance and skill to research and to type up their own program design. They will also find out later on that it is also as equally difficult to type up the right amount of information necessary to complete the program design itself. In preparing a program design, there is that feeling of anxiety and frustration of describing something out of nothing particularly when you have to write about a matter that you have never seen nor done before. To a few who may have actual experiences as a former staff member in a residential care setting, they may have little advantage but having the experience alone is one thing, but preparing a program design, a business plan and setting up the business itself is totally different. Others may have the convenience of hiring the services of a professional consultant/program designer who normally charges between $3,000 to $7,000 per program depending on the type of facility and the complexity of the program to design. So, I wrote this book and included in the exhibit sections a couple of sample program designs that you as a beginner can use as a guide to observe when you write your own program design. Undoubtedly, your own program design will be somewhat different from my sample and so does everyone else but at least you have a general idea on what to discuss in your writing material, right? A fair warning to the reader, you are not the only one who has a copy of my book so, do not make the mistake of just copying the sample from this book word for word. As long as you do not present your program design as if it was copied verbatim from my book, you will do fine.

With the inclusion of sample program designs alone and the helpful tips that are mentioned in this book, you will be saving yourself thousands of dollars and avoid annoying headaches and frustration that you could normally encounter in preparing yourself for the business.

When you read this book, you are theoretically placing yourself ahead of the game just like being transported ahead of time and understanding the business first before you actually make the decision to be in it for the long haul or not. That way, should you decide to finally get in the care-giving business for the first time, you have an idea on what you need to do with the business from day one, how to do it the right way in order to get the business started and running; and of course make a profit as a result of your effort. With the basic knowledge you acquire from reading this book and from other sources, you will feel more confident with your decision whether to continue from this point to the next which is to initiate and implement your plans and to do the suggested steps written in this book.

Should you decide however, to take the easier way which is to just drop the whole thing and go back to your respective jobs or whatever you were doing instead of making this business to work, at least, it would only have cost you a very small fraction of the risk which is practically the cost of this book instead of something else rather than realize later on that the business is not for you.

UNDECIDED YET? Another option for you to consider should you become undecided whether to move forward or to hold off to your plans temporarily is to save more money towards your business. Perhaps, later on you may reconsider in a different time and mind frame. Considering the fact that you might need a substantial amount of money to start this business, it is always wise to think and rethink your plans before committing yourself. There are things to consider when you start a business and some part of it which I am sure you know is planning, finances, experience and commitment in the business.

Another important factor to consider is your available financial resources. You need to know how much money you might need in order to survive the crucial initial stages of the business that is why it is important to prepare a business plan first or hire someone to prepare it for you before doing anything else. With that in mind, contrary to most popular belief, you do not need a lot of cash to establish a residential care facility as it all depends on the type of facility and the clients that you intend to serve. The higher the level of the facility, the more services you must provide. The cost of establishing this business could be started at a bare minimum just enough to get the business started. What is considered as bare minimum? Later on, I will discuss how much money you will need to get started and learn how and where you can get FREE start up funds for your business.

You have to understand that the process could take at least six to eight months or sometimes longer before you can receive your first referral depending on the effort that you put in and your ability to meet the requirements set by your local licensing agencies and your vendorizing agencies. That is why it is a good idea not to quit your day jobs until you feel comfortable that your business is starting to take off or at least more than breaking even.

In getting an appointment with your local fire marshal to come and visit your facility for certification, you have to first submit your program design with your application for a license. Then, community care licensing office will request the marshal to conduct his/her certification visit on your property based on what purpose stated on your application. Perhaps, after you secure your license to operate a facility you might have to wait for another month or two for vendorization by your local placement agencies who will give you the referral for your business. You might also need to evaluate your past experience, your contribution to the business, the support system and the alternative resource that is available to you in order to keep your business running.

You will need to know how much money you have to retain to keep the business alive temporarily while you wait to accommodate your first clients, and of course a full staff on stand-by available and ready to assist the consumers in a short notice should placement agencies refer consumers on an emergency basis.

Reality Check: This resource material will try to paint a picture of the business as realistically as possible but it is up to you, the reader to explore and research more on the information presented as each facility level or design may vary. This book will also give you general ideas to consider, that you may convert into useful tools in your quest to overcome your challenges in establishing your own residential care business.

Financing your business: In this book, you will find suggestions on possible ways to finance the business, important tips on where to get funding, what agencies to approach and how to receive grants from various non-profit and for profit entities and learn ways to get free money for your start up funds.

Establishing your business entity or corporation may pose as a challenge even to an experienced individual. So, in this book you will also find a sample guide in setting up and registering your business entity/corporation with the Secretary of State, which local public agencies to approach, forms to fill and useful tips on what to do to make your business official.

This book will also provide you with a checklist of important things to do when you submit your application for a facility license. It also provides useful tips in getting your facility vendorized in order to receive placement referrals regularly. It has a special section just for those who are interested in responding to a request for a proposal RFP, and lots more.....

To those of you who want to set up their first residential care facility whether it be a Small Family Home, Foster Family Home, Foster Family Agency, Group Home, Transitional Housing Placement Home, An Adult Residential Care Facility, Residential Care Facility for the Elderly and the Chronically Ill; A Day Program, Adult Day Care, Adult Day Health Care, Senior Day Care and Senior Day Health Care Center; the information presented in this book is very useful and is written just for you. So, have fun reading it and enjoy the learning experience.

Good luck in all your plans and go for your dreams. It can only happen if you want it to happen.

So, read on. I look forward to hearing about you and your successes in the near future.... RMS

INTRODUCTION

After reading the basics of starting up a business, perhaps your next question might be.... Do you need to have experience in a residential care setting to be able to get this started? YES, but not necessarily true at all times depending on the type of facility you are considering to establish. Back then, approximately 10 to 15 years ago, anyone can become a residential care facility owner-administrator without any experience at all. But rest assured there were also a lot who failed too soon in the business. But, with the growing demand to upgrade the quality of care services, state and federal bills and regulations were passed elevating the bar of expectation including the requirement that all facilities must have a certified facility administrator who has at least 6 months to one year of experience in the residential care type of setting that the applicant is applying for in order for the application to be processed. However, this should not dampen your spirits from achieving your goal. There are ways to go about it that is why I wrote this book. Realistically, it is also a good idea to at least have a direct experience on the type of business that you are considering, learn what it takes to make it succeed, evaluate how the business is run, and consider the things you need to find out for your self if this is what you really want to do as a business.

However, to those who may lack the experience and the knowledge of the business, you might want to think about hiring someone with the right experience and the knowledge to help establish and to operate the business for a year or so, until you are ready to be on your own. Consider your self under training while being shadowed by your employee-Administrator/Program Director. The requirement may appear to be fair and literally reasonable because, being in a business that requires considerable amount of investment, patience and time, definitely, you need to know what it takes to make it work accordingly otherwise, all the effort you exert will become useless. The experience requirement is similar to a famous saying, "what comes first, the egg or the chicken".

How can you acquire the experience if the job is limited only to those with experience? Well, there are ways to respond to the issue and sometimes, you will find the right answer in few unexpected ways. To those who simply do not have the required experience but may have deeper pockets and can afford to buy more time, consider looking for other alternative solutions and here are a couple of possible suggestions:

(a). **Volunteer in a facility**. Since the whole process may take at least six (6) to eight (8) months to complete from initial application to final visit/inspection of the facility and issuance of a provisional license, you might have enough time to volunteer or work at a facility to gain the much needed experience while you are waiting completion of the application process.

(b). **Invite experienced individual(s) to contribute to your Company/Business and share the benefits of co-ownership**.

(c). **Hire an Experienced Program Director or Administrator.** There are literally a handful of certified facility administrators readily available out there whom you can sign up for the job in a flash. They may be able to represent you for a good cause or at a reasonable price.

Time is Always Right

Excuses come easy. If you really want your own business, there is only one challenge that you will struggle with at the beginning... PROCRASTINATION. Your ability to delay your plans to another date and time will only slow you down in an instant. You can come up with all the excuses if you want to and procrastinate as you watch someone else reap the benefit that should have been yours to keep. One thing is certain, my friend, no one will knock on your door to help lead you to your success, nobody else but you. So, let's face it. Some of us will never be able to start up this business for one way or another due to lots of reasons such as fear of the unknown, health, money, etc... If that is how you think, your dreams will be nothing more than just a mere fantasy or an illusion. You will hope for it, think about it, and come up with hundred reasons why you can not do it.

Be positive. Whatever it is that you want for your self, your business will need more from you than just to dream on. But, then again, you may be one of the few who are ready to get started in this business but do not have a slightest idea on what to do next after the orientation. Perhaps you may have had the experience in the past as a care provider or in management and know what the business is all about, but is that enough? Maybe it's your first time but you have set aside all your fear or doubt and anxious to get it started already. It is all up to you. Why not try to go through a simplified Acid Test which basically will help you make your own realization if the business is for you. You need to answer the questions as honestly and sincerely as possible.

The Acid Test

Will you enjoy this business of caring for others?
Will you do your best effort to make it work no matter what it takes?
Will you personally manage the business or with a group?
Will your earnings from the business meet your expectations?
Will you be able to financially keep the business going for a long term?

These five points will answer the question of what you can do for the business and in return what the business can do for you. In any relationship, there must be cohesive relationship between the business owner and the enterprise and both must blend to create a workable status and it only happens when all scores are high on all key points raised in the test. Consider them one by one, then, read on.

Most people think that money is their number one priority in getting into this business. If I were you, I'll put that at the bottom of the list and place the psychological rewards on top. When you enjoy the business that you are in, success and money will naturally come in abundance, but does not work quite well in reverse. If one happen to make serious money in a business he does not enjoy, the essence of the challenge becomes worthless. Getting into a business of your own is not that easy at all. You must first check out the business. Create a business plan and a marketing plan to help you understand the business. Ask other people who are in the business or those who has been through it before. Base on those observations and research perhaps you can make an intelligent decision. If you have a job, it is always a good idea to keep it temporarily until you get the facility business going or at least get it up and started already before quitting your regular jobs.

When you are in the right business, there is a thrill to it all. You will see the business being born and watch it grow before your very eyes. You will nurse it through the survival stage, navigate it to its apex and when you are finished, you will probably let it take its own course from there on.

Check Out Your Management Mentality

What type of management mentality do you need to start up with the business? First, since you are starting up on a budget, consider your self at the bottom of the payroll as the only staff member for now who will do all the hard work that is needed in the facility. Once the business picks up and have more than two consumers (customers) in your home/facility, then perhaps you might need someone to help you on a consistent basis. As your consumer population grows, then you might need to start exercising your management talent.

Comparing your self to someone who may have deeper pockets and can afford to hire a staff at the beginning, your challenge may be a little bit different but the outcome shall remain the same. So, do not feel bad at all.

"What do you know or need to know in running a "board and care" facility business?" It is amazing to observe how many people who have never worked in a residential care setting before, but with enthusiasm and sheer optimism they impulsively fork in their hard earned savings into the business. What's more amazing is that some people actually make it. Call it luck or whatever, but in reality most of it is hard work and proper planning. Experience alone does not magically transform yourself into an excellent manager. Let this be your guide… if you do not have the help, the experience in this type of business and proper planning, do not attempt to open the business right away. You might want to hold on until you are ready and have obtained valuable "hands-on" experience and knowledge perhaps as an employee at the beginning or at least hire an experienced manager to help show you the ropes of the business.

You might also have to moonlight for a little while flipping burgers and fries at a food station while you pick up the experience and perhaps sacrifice some income for a few months in exchange for the experience that you need. How many of us are willing to do that? But it will be much worth it in the long term compared to what you will expect from running a business that you know nothing about.

Consider these options:

1. Get the experience that is needed.

2. Hire an experienced staff and a qualified administrator to temporarily show you the way of the business.

3. Partner with a group of reliable individuals who have the expertise or experience in the business.

4. Become a mentor or be mentored by someone who knows the business.

5. Hire an experienced consultant to guide you through.

Another way to approach the challenge is to tighten your belt and not to expect so much at first. No one can actually predict how successful the business will be as the start up year is always the most difficult one. It is purely up to you. As you go along with the process, you will discover for your self that this undertaking is not really that difficult at all. There are hundred ways to keep the business in shape as it could require a lot of flexibility from your end to keep it going. In my experience helping other people in getting their business up and running, I observed a lot of successful start-ups who had to force themselves at the beginning to keep their "part time jobs" even if they have their business going already just to allow the income to flow within the business. Others lived delicately on cash reserves while others may have other different resources. Whether or not you have income independent of the business, you must be able to flex the business a little to make it work effectively.

What is the bottom line?

What does this business really mean to you? You need to do a self-assessment. It is never easy to be objective when you are asking the tough questions about your self. But when you know your goal and needs; strengths and limitations, you practically have a better understanding of what you will go through.

It is hard for me to understand why people start their own business and then complain that opportunities do not exist. More opportunities exist in the business today than ever before, despite rumors of pending moratorium, possible suspension of license issuances to brand new care facilities or the limitation on the number of pending vendors or accreditation, etc... Common sense might help you understand that the population is growing and so is the need to accommodate the growing needs and services. Perhaps, there may be valid reasons behind the temporary suspension of the issuance of accreditation or licenses to facilities (if any), therefore, it is always a good idea to first secure reliable information from your local licensing agency and other placement agencies before you start making your big plans. It is also a good plan to get things up and running as far as paper work and processing is concerned while there are moratoriums so that once the hold is lifted, you are already positioned to a point that will give you flexible options to consider when the opportunity arises. Depending on how you look at it. To some who are half-hearted in this business, they may find the moratorium an opportunity to just hold off to their dream and to go back to their jobs or whatever they were doing. Despite the rumors of budget cuts and moratorium spells, there is no reason why this business should be placed on the cutting table. Realistically, somehow, someone has to take care of the consumers needs in any way.

Current businesses may not have sufficient resources to accommodate the growing demand. With possible over supply of the average board and care homes on certain areas, licensing and vendorizing agencies do not have better options but to increase the bar of expectation in the quality standard of the services and demand for new and unique types of services in facilities thereby resulting in the provision of a cost effective service delivery system. The bottom line is that, there is a need for a new service facility all the time no matter what, no matter when and no matter how.

How Others Found Success in this Business.

Do you think you have the right business approach? The answer is not found in this book. If I had the foolproof crystal ball I would be too busy sipping my favorite drink on ice in Peter Island somewhere in the Caribbean to tell you the truth. Nobody else (except for the fortune tellers who pretend to have all the right answers) can tell you what you want to hear. Part of the challenge in this business is to find out for yourself. It bears its similarities to gambling with calculated risk. In order for us to have a general idea about the business and how the business shall be in a few months down the road, it is always a good idea to prepare a business plan which shall serve as a roadmap to your success. Just like in the old saying …"it is always good to plan because if you fail to plan, you already planned to fail". Establish a business plan and try to understand the business; try to pin point as to what your financial situation shall be like; formulate "what if" scenarios as they are a good guide in better understanding the business. Creating possible financial scenarios will help you get some ideas on what to do on the good side of the business up to the worse scenario if it does occur.

Flexibility is one factor to consider especially when you are just starting fresh. It includes your ability to flex your expenses, personal income, work schedule and of course your role as staff member/administrator/owner. You also need to maintain a mind set that you are not just in the business of providing care services, you are also in investments and real estate.

Gross revenues should not cloud your mission to primarily provide a service to the people you promised to serve. Staffing is another important key to remember. You must have good people, and choose the ones with proven records of quality performance. Last but not the least, you have to have a hands on management and not allow someone else to run your business. You must be on top of every aspect of the operation of the business. You must not rely solely on your staff members. Remember, it is just a job to them, you are the licensee and your business is on the line.

Are you ready for this? All right! Now that you are, LET'S GET STARTED.

In this book, you will be provided with an important checklist of the things that a new provider may need to complete in order to initially get the business set-up. Later on, the checklist topics will be explained in general detail as to what needs to be done on every stage of the process. You need to understand that the guide being presented here may vary from county to county or from state to another but the basic requirements in setting up a residential care business remain the same whether you are in California or in another state. Each and everyone of you may have different challenges and unique situations when you bought this book, so you must adjust accordingly and only use the information which applies to your particular situation. At some point, a number of you may have met a few of the requirements already, so as long as you accomplish most if not all of the requirements, you will do fine. Each facility type as well as individual situations may require different documentations but generally, the documentation process and requirements remain the same and all of it are enumerated in this book. If you have a different situation when you purchased this book, it is a good idea to read thru the applicable stages and try to accomplish as much documentations as possible to meet the requirement.

Chapter 1: UNDERSTANDING THE RESIDENTIAL CARE BUSINESS

THE FACILITY: A Perspective.

I. Learning the Business.

For those who are starting up the business for the very first time, the most important thing to do now is to learn a little bit more about the business, its history, the past, present and future of the business. This chapter will also give you an idea on what your chances of success are in the business and is it feasible or is it really worth it for you to consider the business?

The business of caring have grown considerably today compared to what it was 15 to 20 years ago. The simplest concept of a mom and pop type of operation years ago has now grown so big that it has become one of the most promising start-up businesses in the nation today. Years ago, facilities that are involved in this caring environment are mostly institutional and clinical in setting. There were a very few that were residential care facility setting typically in a home-like environment just like the home where you and I normally live. With recent changes in federal and state regulations on health care, the business of caring has been altered from a simple to a more complex business partly due to the revolutionary changes and trends in the health care industry.

There is no written chronicle as to how the residential care business actually evolved. Perhaps there was none at the time when this book was written but there are some acceptable theories from different agency representatives which are reflected in this book. Please bear in mind that the theory arose purely from conjecture and is not necessarily conclusive.

Brief history of the business can be related to unconfirmed records dating back in the early years when this beautiful nation which we now call the United States of America was initially inhabited by the native Indians of North America. The discovery of the new world resulted in the influx of other nationalities and cultures from other foreign lands. Most of the things that were introduced in this great nation were cultures, laws and tradition, beliefs, practices, religion and norms of our early immigrants. With the revolution of a new order, it brought about the conversion to a more complex lifestyle which eventually brought us to our current socio-politico-economic environment which we now consider the American lifestyle.

Looking at our socio-cultural evolution in retrospect, our current social problem is a result of our past experiences starting from the date of our initial migration. Our forefathers and peoples before them brought in their cultures and tradition which back then was the norm. But as the years went by, some cultural practices slowly deteriorated to become part of the social problems we have today. A good example was the use of punishment or the infliction of bodily harm, discipline or in some religions as a way to drive the demon from their bodies, the use of medications to help ease pain or cause hallucination was socially and medically acceptable and was even introduced as refreshments up until such time that those practices were declared illegal and unlawful. All these related issues resulted in the contribution to the social problems of the current time, which include abuse, neglect, developmental disabilities, mental illness, abnormalities of the human body that affect somatic cells or tissues of every organ system. The people who looked and acted differently back then were left at home or in mental hospitals, tied up in their beds, but living in fear of abusive treatment and isolation from the society. Now, our society has matured and become very supportive of the developmentally challenged. This evolution we can now attribute to the creation of laws and regulations which led to the establishment of public and private agencies that protect and advocate for those individuals and families affected by these social problems.

These agencies we now call the Department of Health and Human Services, Department of Social Services, Department of Mental Health, Department of Aging, etc… These agencies with the support from federal funding and the community helped create entities that support their mission statement which led to the establishment of hospitals, mental health institutions, Adult Protective Services, Child Protective Services, etc.. With the passing of several sponsored bills and legislations, it further led to the creation of private and public care homes, group homes etc.… where we as members of the society are able to monitor and look after the interest of the less fortunate, particularly the children, the developmentally disabled, the mentally ill and the aged. That is why sometime in the early 1970's and 80's led to the mushrooming of facilities that care for individuals in need of the services and such facilities we know now as **licensed residential care facilities** also known in layman's terms as **board and care homes.**

With the passing of the various welfare bills advocating for the increased protection of the rights of children, the developmentally disabled and the aging citizenry, there have been significant changes in the health care industry. All these changes have been focused on the improvement of the deplorable quality of care among facilities. These either challenged and encouraged facility owners and operators to accept the radical changes and make necessary adjustments, or on the other hand discouraged and rooted out the ones that were not meeting the standards and expectations set by the regulating agencies. There will be a discussion on these important changes as we go through the succeeding chapters. Contrary to what a lot of people think, the board and care home business is not easy to establish and let alone make a lot of money from it in a very short time. It requires a considerable amount of patience, perseverance and a lot of genuine unconditional love of people in need of personal care services. It is quite ironic to note that the care providers sometimes have a closer relationship with their clients more than they have with their own families as they technically spend more time on their jobs out of necessity and dedication. Obviously, it has something to do with the economics of the job initially and eventually incline towards the humanitarian side of the care. Sometimes it is a wonder to think why people actually get into this business despite of the fact that it could take time before one can actually recoups his investment. There is a considerable amount of risk involved and sometimes the amount of compensation is not enough in comparison to the responsibility that it requires. Such risks include the high probability of verbal and physical abuse from the residents, the possibility of contracting various forms of diseases, habits, the pressure from the regulating agencies, frustrations from the justice system; not to forget the possibility of criminal sanctions for serious allegation and a multitude of challenges on behind-the-scenes of managing a residential care business. If somehow you feel unsure about what you are getting into, this is the best time to back out now or you may choose to step up to the plate and face the challenge. Focus on your objective if this is what you really want. No doubt the business can be easily learned and may be financially rewarding, but nothing can place monetary value to the type of satisfaction that you can receive for the efforts that you contribute in helping towards the improvement of the quality of life of people in need of help. There will be instances when discouragement settles in because despite of all the efforts exerted in this business, you might see futile outcomes. Results of one's contributions are eventually observed on a long term basis and in small increments. Remember that you can only do so much on a limited time and with very limited amount of resources. In frustrating times like this, just remember to ask GOD for "help to change the things that can be changed, accept those that you can not, and to have the humility and the knowledge to understand the difference".

As a care provider, there is a standard of care expected from you by the County, the State and Federal agencies who entrust you with the life of people in need of help, individuals whom they think are safe in your hands. They will constantly monitor your activities, the funds that they entrust to you. Strict regulations, laws and other guidelines will be passed to make sure that providers will do what they committed to do. All around the country, there are thousands of care facilities out there that are currently in operation and yours will be just like one of them. With the increasing number of facilities available, each state and county may have their own set of guidelines in granting a facility license to operate and in order to remain in business. In some counties, they are limiting the number of facilities within their jurisdiction to prevent over supply of particular services in certain areas. However, with the ever-growing population in the next decade, and the fusion of cultural changes in our society brought about by the advancement of technology and evolution in lifestyle, families will always be in the midst of all these whirl wind of changes. These changes will definitely bring about stress in families and those who can not cope up will seek the assistance of the various state, county and federal agencies, who will in turn secure the support of health care providers like yourself. Therefore, if we are to speculate on the future of the residential care business, it is undoubtedly a bright and promising one.

II. What is long-term care?

In the past, when we talk about long-term care, most people think of custodial care only for the elderly in a nursing homes or skilled nursing facilities. As we learn through the years that long-term care as we know today includes a wide variety of settings and services which are available to meet people's special needs not only for the elderly but will also include meeting the needs of children, adults and seniors with medical, behavioral, psycho-social and developmental disabilities or self help needs. Between 1990 and 2020, there are approximately 87 Million Americans who will be retiring and not to mention those individuals young and not so young who will receive medical treatment and would be recovering from surgery may stay in a sub-acute care facility instead of a hospital. A stroke or accident victim can receive nursing care and speech, physical and occupational therapy at a skilled nursing facility. It could also be someone who requires assistance with activities of daily living such as dressing, feeding and bathing, but does not need 24-hour nursing, may choose a residential care facility setting where services are relatively affordable. Other options include respite care and adult day health care to ease the burden on family caregivers, special Alzheimer's programs, services for persons with developmental disabilities, mental health care, and home and community based care.

III. Who needs long-term care?

There will be two out of every five Americans who will need long-term care at some point in their lives. Seniors are the fastest growing segment of our population and are the heaviest users of long-term health care services. In California, the elderly population (age 65+) is expected to grow more than twice as fast as the total population. The elderly age group will have an average increase of 112% during the period 1990-2020.

More than any other socio-economic group, women are disproportionately affected by long-term care. The reason behind this lies in the fact that women live longer than men and thus, are more likely to develop the functional ailments that require long-term care services. Two-thirds of residents in long-term care facilities are women.

Romwell Martinez Sabeniano, MBA.HCM

There are several other factors contribute to the need for long-term care. Families are geographically scattered. Time, travel, expenses and other responsibilities make it nearly impossible to provide the care to individuals with disabilities and older family members need. In addition, the primary caregivers in most families are women, and today more women work outside their home. Although long-term care services are mostly used by the elderly; young adults, children, and even infants use long term care services due to chronic illness, disability or accident.

IV. What are the different types of long-term care services available?

A. Home and Community-Based Care

1. Community Care Facilities: Community care facilities provide 24-hour non-medical residential care to children, adults and seniors with developmental disabilities including seniors and adults without disabilities unable to care for themselves and those with mental illness. This category may include the care for high risk-assaultive children in a group home setting.

- Regulation: Licensed by Dept of Social Services, Community Care Licensing Division.
- Payment: Funding through home and community-based Medi-Cal waiver program, Foster Care Rates Bureau, Dept. of Social Services, Regional Center funding for the developmentally disabled.

   1. Small Family Homes (SFH)
   2. Foster Family Homes (FFH)
   3. Foster Family Agency (FFA)
   4. Transitional Housing (TH)
   5. Group Homes (GH)
   6. Adult Residential Care Facility (ARF)
   7. Residential Care Facility for the Elderly (RCFE)
   8. Residential Care Facility for the Chronically Ill (RCFCI)
   9. Adult Day Care Facility (ADCF) / Social Day Care (SDC)

An Easy Guide On How to Establish Your First Residential Care Facility

In order to simplify our discussion on the business, the book will be limiting its scope on understanding the above enumerated facilities known as community care facilities.

2. Congregate Housing: Housing with a common living area and non-medical support services to meet basic needs of older people.

- Regulation: Dept of Social Services, Community Care Licensing Division.
- Payment: Grants provided through the Federal Government (Housing & Urban Development). Some funding through SSI/SSP for those eligible.

3. Home Health Care: Home health care provides medically-oriented care for acute or chronic illness in the patient's home, usually as a follow-up to acute or other facility discharge.

- Regulation: Licensed and Medicare and Medi-Cal certified by DHS.
- Payment: Funded primarily through Medicare, with limited coverage through Medi-Cal, private insurance and private payments.

4. Hospice: Hospice provides care and support for terminally ill people and their families. It can be provided in a facility setting or at home.

- Regulation: Hospice license required for in-home care. Dual license required in a facility setting. Medicare certification required for Medicare or Medi-Cal payments.
- Payment: Funded through Medicare, Medi-Cal, private insurance and private payments.

5. Personal care services: Personal care services are provided for people who need assistance with daily living but do not require nursing.

- Regulation: No separate license required.

- Payment: Primarily funded through In-Home Supportive Services for those eligible. Some Medi-Cal, for those eligible, and private payments.

6. Respite care: Respite care provides short term inpatient or home care delivered to an elderly person as a substitute for their regular caregiver.

- Regulation: No separate license required of existing licensed providers.
- Payment: Funding through home and community based waiver and the Department of Aging.

B. Facility-Based Care:

1. Residential-Care Facilities for the Elderly (RCFEs). Assisted living facilities provide personal care and safe housing for people who may need supervision for medication and assistance with daily living but who do not require 24-hour nursing care.

- Regulation: Licensed by Dept. of Social Services, Community Care Licensing Division.
- Payment: Primarily through private payments. Nearly 30% of RCFE residents rely on SSI/SSP non-medical out-of-home grants.

2. Continuing Care Retirement Communities (CCRCs). It includes three levels of care: independent, assisted living and nursing care. CCRCs require an entrance fee paid by the applicant upon admission and includes services for more than one year and up to the lifetime of the resident.

- Regulation: Licensed by Dept. of Social Services, Continuing Care Contracts Branch. Skilled nursing level licensed by the Dept. of Health Services.
- Payment: Private Payment

3. Intermediate-Care Facilities (ICF's). These facilities provide room and board along with regular medical, nursing, social and rehabilitative services for people not capable of full independent living.

- Regulation: Licensed by Health Care Licensing and paid thru Medi-Cal and/or Medicare certified by DHS.
- Payment: Funding primarily provided by Medi-Cal. Some funding through Medicare and private payment.

4. Intermediate-Care Facilities for the Developmentally Disabled (ICF/DDs). This is known at the federal level as ICF's/MR (mental retardation), these facilities provide services for people of all ages with mental retardation and/or developmental disabilities. ICF/DD's have 16 or more beds; ICF/DD-H (habilitative) and N's (nursing) have 15 or fewer beds and average six beds in a home setting.

- Regulation: Licensed thru Health Care Licensing and Medi-Cal certified by DHS. The Department of Developmental Services and Regional Centers are responsible for placement and quality assurance.
- Payment: Nearly 100% Medi-Cal.

5. Institutes for Mental Health (SNF/STPs). Designated in California as "special treatment programs," these facilities provide extended treatment programs for people of all ages with chronic mental-health problems; many of the clients are younger than 65. Specialized staff serves clients in a secured environment.

- Regulation: Licensed and Medi-Cal certified by Department of Health Services DHS. Local mental health departments are responsible for placement and program content.
- Payment: A combination of state and county funding.

6. Skilled Nursing Facilities (SNF's). SNF's, or nursing homes/convalescent hospitals, provide comprehensive nursing care for chronically ill or short-term residents of all ages, along with rehabilitation and specialized medical programs.

- Regulation: Licensed and Medi-Cal and/or Medicare certified by the California Department of Health Services (DHS).
- Payment: Funded primarily by Medi-Cal. Some funding provided through Medicare, managed care and private payment.

7. Sub-acute Care Facilities. Specialized units often in a distinct part of a nursing facility, sub-acute-care facilities focus on intensive rehabilitation, complex wound care and post-surgical recovery for residents of all ages who no longer need the level of care found in a hospital.

- Regulation: Licensed and Medi-Cal and/or Medicare certified by DHS.
- Payment: Funded primarily by Medi-Cal. Some funding through Medicare, managed care and private payment.

If we will discuss each and every facility mentioned, it could take us more time than what is necessary and it could become too confusing to read at the beginning. So, in order to prevent you from experiencing information overload, this book will focus its discussion on residential care facilities which our business will be based on and they are the following:

Different types of Facilities available through Community Care Licensing?

1. Small Family Homes (SFH)
2. Foster Family Homes (FFH)
3. Foster Family Agency (FFA)
4. Transitional Housing (TH)
5. Group Homes (GH)
6. Adult Residential Care Facility (ARF)
7. Residential Care Facility for the Elderly (RCFE)
8. Residential Care Facility for the Chronically Ill (RCFCI)
9. Adult Day Care Facility (ADCF) / Social Day Care (SDC)

As a matter of common practice, the manner of establishing any of the above-mentioned facilities are very similar to each other. If there is a slight difference, it shall be easily observed depending on the specific type of facility. The higher the standard of care and service expectations there is on the particular type of facility, the more requirement there is that is expected to be met. But, generally the procedures, the steps and guidelines in establishing any residential care facility business are very similar if not oddly identical. So, do not feel confused regardless of the type of facility you are considering.

The first five categories of facilities namely small family home, foster family home, foster family agency, transitional housing and group home involves placement for children who are victims of family abuse, neglect and the family's inability to care for their children. This temporary living arrangement where children will live in a family like setting often times with another group of children from different families in a 6 bed home supervised on a 24 hour non-medical basis operated by either a mom and dad type of setting or by a staff representing a private or non-profit organization directly responsible for the care and supervision. Most if not all of the placements in these homes are undertaken as a result of a mandate from the family court advocating for the rights and interest of families particularly the children.

SMALL FAMILY HOME (SFH)

Provides 24 hour-a-day care in the licensee's family residence for six or fewer children who are abused and neglected; mentally disordered, developmentally disabled, or physically handicapped, and who require special care and supervision as a result of such disabilities. Majority of these homes are situated in single family residences or apartment units typically run by a mom-dad and their adult children who themselves comprises the staff that takes care of the residents. The placement is either for a short term or a long term depending on the reason why the resident is placed. It is similar to the set up of a foster family home but the difference is that it is operated on its own, for its own and by its own. In order to become a small family home business operator, one must secure licensing from the local Community Care Licensing office of the Department of Social and secure vendorization from the placing agencies such as the Child Protective Services, Regional Center, Dept. of Health, Dept. of Mental Health etc... If the individual is a child or an adult with developmental disabilities who has specialized needs, Regional Center is the placing agency that will provide vendorization placements and licensing will be authorized by Health Care Licensing.

FOSTER FAMILY HOME (FFH)

Provides 24-hour care and supervision in a family type setting in the licensee's family residence for no more than six (6) children. Care is provided to children who have been removed from the home due to neglect or abuse, children who require special health or who are mentally disordered, developmentally disabled, physically handicapped, and who require care and supervision due to disabilities. Similar to a small family home in terms of its general operation but the difference is that foster family homes are run by families but are operated by a foster family agency that registers and places the residents to individual family's homes and monitor their progress on a regular basis. Placement is either for a short term or a long term until the child turns 18 years old and able to live independently. To those who are interested in becoming a care-provider or as a foster parent, one must secure accreditation from a foster family agency that is provided with a license to operate a foster family agency and receive placements from the children's agencies that will place the children in foster family homes.

FOSTER FAMILY AGENCY (FFA)

A non-profit organization engaged in the recruiting, certifying, and training of, and providing professional support to certified parents, or in finding homes for placement of children for temporary or permanent care who require that level of care as an alternative to a group home setting. This is the agency directly responsible to the placing agency (typically the Dept. of Children and Family Services, Child Protective Services etc…)

TRANSITIONAL HOUSING (TH)

An extension program intended for children coming from group homes who by their ages (exceeding 17 years of age) and by maturity are almost ready for emancipation but are still in need of a short term support from government agencies. These adolescent children are provided with housing and support until they achieve self-reliance and independence. A typical transitional housing is situated in apartment complexes and single family homes where the child-resident lives responsibly with other residents in a home like setting where they learn to transition into adulthood. It is a way for a child who is used to living in a group home setting yet too young or totally unprepared to live independently on his/her own. Sometimes even if a child turns 18 and comes from a group home setting but if he/she is deemed unprepared to live alone, the agency takes care of his/her needs up to the age 22.

This is one of the latest "in demand" sector of the residential care business. A good number of my former students requested information on this program and in response to those numerous requests, I have included in the book a discussion on this subject which will be found later on in this chapter.

GROUP HOME (GH)

A group home provides 24-hour non-medical care and supervision to children in a structured environment. Services are provided, at least in part, either by the owner/licensee and or by staff employed by the licensee. Group home licensees are responsible for the care and supervision of the children placed in the group home. Group homes are licensed by the California Department of Social Services **(CDSS)**, Community Care Licensing Division (CCLD). CCLD monitors group homes by making unannounced visits at least once per year and as frequently as necessary to make sure that the facilities meet the regulations.

The children are placed in the group homes by the county social services and probation departments (which makes the highest number of placements of children in these residential facilities), county mental health agencies and regional centers. Parents, private individuals or families may also place children for whom they have legal custody whereby such placements are called voluntary placements.

Assuming at this stage that you have decided to put up a group home. Then, you have to determine what type of children you would be willing to accept as your clients. There are four different types of children that are placed in group homes which will be discussed later on in the succeeding chapters.

ADULT RESIDENTIAL FACILITY (ARF)

This is a residential care facility of any capacity (typically 4-6 bed) that provides 24 hour non-medical care for adults, between ages 18-59 years, who are not able to provide for their own daily needs, the physically handicapped, developmentally disabled, and/or mentally disordered. Adult residential care facilities are either operated by a family or by staff representing a placement organization.

RESIDENTIAL CARE FACILITY FOR THE ELDERLY (RCFE)

Facility of any capacity that provide non-medical care to persons 60 years of age and over or persons under 60 with compatible needs; elderly residents requiring varying levels and intensities of care and supervision and protective supervision or personal care; elderly who may be frail and/or disabled, and cannot, or do not desire to take care of their own daily needs.

RESIDENTIAL CARE FACILITY FOR THE CHRONICALLY ILL (RCFCI)

This is a facility with a licensed capacity of 25 or less, that provides care and supervision to adults who have persistent terminal illness, Acquired Immune Deficiency Syndrome (AIDS), or the Human-Immunodeficiency Virus (HIV).

ADULT DAY CARE FACILITY (ADCF) / SOCIAL DAY CARE (SDCF)

Facility of any capacity that provides activity programs for frail adults and elderly and developmentally disabled individuals, and / or mentally disordered in a day care setting.

TRANSITIONAL HOUSING

WHAT IS TRANSITIONAL HOUSING AND HOW COME YOU HAVE NEVER HEARD OF IT BEFORE?

Transitional Housing Placement THP is one of the hottest business potential that one might consider as an alternative. It is one of the most unpopular types of residential care business available simply because not a lot of people actually know much about it. It is observed that out of 50 residential care facility owners there are perhaps only less than 2% who are in transitional housing business. One of the reasons being is that transitional housing is fairly new compared to the rest of the residential care businesses known to many. With the growing population of children from group homes for high risk and at risk children and other similar types of facilities where the individual turns 18 years of age and has proven potentials for independent living whether developmentally disabled or not, transitional housing is another alternative setting to look into. The property structure commonly used in most of these type of facilities are leased to own duplexes-triplexes, single family homes or apartment-condominium complexes where adult individuals or groups of individuals coming from the Social Services system, Dept. of Developmental Services, Dept. of Mental Health, Dept. of Corrections, Regional Center, Dept. of Probation, etc... attempt to transition from adolescent life to responsible adulthood. As these individuals attempt to transition to live on their own but are still emotionally, psychologically, developmentally unprepared, this facility program will be able to assist them in attaining their personal objective of self-dependence by providing temporary housing and programming that is geared towards the accomplishment of their goal to eventually live independently. The programming environment provided in these homes are very limited in their structure as the adults are treated or supposed to be treated as responsible adult individuals.

Here are some general guidelines on Transitional Housing also known as Transitional Housing Placement Facility:

Transitional housing placement facility means either of the following:

(a). A community care facility licensed by the State Department of Social Services pursuant to Section 1559.110 of the Health and Safety Code to provide transitional housing opportunities to persons at least 16 years old, and not more than 18 years old unless they satisfy the requirements of Health and Safety Code Section 11403, who are in out-of-home placement under the supervision of the county department of social services or the county probation department, and who are participating in an independent living program. Welfare and Institutions Code Section 11403 provides in part: A child who is in foster care and receiving aid pursuant to this chapter and who is attending high school or the equivalent level of vocational or technical training on a full-time basis prior to his or her 18th birthday, may continue to receive aid following his or her 18th birthday so long as the child continues to reside in foster care placement, remains otherwise eligible for AFDC-FC payments, and continues to attend high school or the equivalent level of vocational or technical training on a full-time basis and the child may reasonably be expected to complete the educational or training program before his or her 19th birthday. Aid shall be provided to such an individual by both the careprovider and the agency responsible for the foster care placement who signs a mutual agreement, (if the individual is capable of making an informed agreement) which documents the continued need for out-of-home placement."

Transitional Housing Placement Program services shall include any of the following setting:

1. Condominium with an adult employee of the provider.

2. Traditional housing placement program in which one or more participants live in an apartment, single-family dwelling or;

3. Programs in which a participant lives independently in an apartment, single-family dwelling, or condominium rented or leased by the provider located in a building in which one or more adult employees of the provider reside and provide supervision.

4. Programs in which a participant lives independently in an apartment, single-family dwelling, or condominium rented or leased by a provider under the supervision of the provider if the State Department of Social Services provides approval.

A transitional housing placement facility that serves only eligible youth over 18 years of age who have emancipated from the foster care system provided that the facility has been certified to provide transitional housing services by the appropriate county social services or probation department, and has obtained a local fire clearance. No later than June 30, 2002, the department shall establish certification standards and procedures in consultation with the County Welfare Directors Association, the California Youth Connection, the county probation departments, and provider representatives. The certification standards shall include, but not be limited to, a criminal background check of transitional housing providers and staff.

The facility must have a current license which shall be posted in a prominent, publicly accessible location in the administrative office of the licensee. A photocopy of the current license shall be retained in the THPF staff residential unit, if applicable.

The residents of a THPF participant living unit shall be limited to the THPF participant, children of participants, THPF employees and their children, if applicable, and ex-participants approved by the licensee, and authorized by the Department's Community Care Licensing Division, to remain in the THPF Unit.

Prior to applying for a license, and in a county that has Department - approved THPF plan, the applicant must submit to the county department of social services or the county probation department a program plan that meets the criteria outlined in the county THPF plan.

The application shall be filed with the licensing agency designated to serve the THPF proposed geographic area of service. An applicant can be licensed to operate a THPF only in counties that have a Department approved THPF plan. If a county does not have a Department-approved THPF plan the THPF provider may provide services in that county only if the provider has:

(a). A host county letter authorizing the THPF provider to provide services in that county; and a license in an adjacent county that does have a Department-approved THPF plan.

(b). The application shall contain a Certificate of Approval from either the county department of social services or the county probation department, approving the applicant's plan of operation. The Certificate of Approval shall verify that the plan of operation meets the criteria outlined in the county THPF plan and includes the provisions of Welfare and Institutions Code Sections 16522-16522.1 as specified in Health and Safety Code Section 1559.115 and Welfare and Institutions Code Section 16522.1.

No applicant shall be issued a license...unless the county department of social services or the county probation department, in the county where the license will be issued, has certified the program as described in Section 16522.1 of the Welfare and Institutions Code. In order to be licensed under this regulation, an applicant shall obtain certification from the county department of social services or the county probation department that the facility program provides all of the following:

(1). Admission criteria for participants in the program, including, but not limited to, consideration of the applicant's age, previous placement history, delinquency history, history of drug or alcohol abuse, current strengths, level of education, mental health history, medical history, prospects for successful participation in the program and work experience.

(2). The department shall review the admission criteria to ensure that the criteria are sufficient to protect participants and that they do not discriminate on the basis of race, gender, sexual orientation, or disability.

(3). Strict employment criteria that will include a consideration of the employee's age, drug or alcohol history, and experience in working with persons in this age group.

(4). A training program designed to primarily educate employees who work directly with participants about the characteristics of persons in this age group placed in long-term care settings, and designed to ensure that these employees are able to adequately supervise and counsel participants and to provide them with training in independent living skills.

An Easy Guide On How to Establish Your First Residential Care Facility

(5). A detailed plan for monitoring the placement of persons under the licensee's care.

(6). A contract between the participating person and the licensee that specifically sets out the requirements for each party, and in the Regulations.

(7). An allowance to be provided to each participant in the program. In the case of a participant living independently, this allowance shall be sufficient for the participant to purchase food and other necessities.

(8). A system for payment for utilities, telephone, and rent.

(9) Policies regarding all of the following:

- (a). Education requirements.
- (b). Work expectations.
- (c). Savings requirements.
- (d). Personal safety.
- (e). Visitors including, but not limited to visitation by the placement agency.
- (f). Emergencies.
- (g). Medical problems.
- (h). Disciplinary measures.
- (i). Childcare.
- (j). Pregnancy.
- (k). Curfew.
- (l). Apartment cleanliness.
- (m). Use of utilities and telephone.
- (n). Budgeting.
- (o). Decorating of apartments.
- (p). Cars.
- (q). Lending or borrowing money.
- (r). Unauthorized purchases.
- (s). Dating.
- (t). Grounds for termination that may include, but shall not be limited to, illegal activities or harboring runaways.
- (u). Apartment furnishings, and a policy on disposition of the furnishings when the resident participant completes the program.

(v). Evaluation of the participant's progress in the program and reporting to the placing agency.

Prior to approval of supervised THPFs in a county, the department shall approve a plan submitted by the county's independent living program that includes assurances that the independent living program shall participate actively in the screening of candidates for this program and shall assist the licensed agency in the supervision of clients participating in the program. The THPF shall secure and maintain for each THPF participant living unit any fire clearance required by and approved by the fire authority having jurisdiction. The THPF shall request a fire clearance for the THPF participant living unit prior to residence of a non-ambulatory individual.

The plan of operation shall contain the following:

(a). The non-ambulatory individual may be the participant, ex-participants approved by the licensee and authorized by the licensing agency to remain in the apartment, the child of a participant living in the units.

(b). The licensee shall provide the licensing agency the business telephone number and the 24-hour emergency telephone number of the THPF licensee or designee.

(c). Complete job descriptions of all THPF employees, including number of staff, classification, qualifications and duties, information regarding lines of authority and staff responsibilities.

A comprehensive program statement including:

1. Goals of the THPF.

2. Description of the youth to be served.

3. Admission criteria for THPF participants, as specified in Welfare and Institutions Code.

4. Staff training plan shall include the following:

(a). Detailed plan for monitoring the THPF participants.

(b). Procedures for responding to complaints and emergencies on a 24-hour basis.

(c). Training new employees.

(d). Ongoing training.

(e). Training topics.

(f). Qualifications of the trainer.

5. Contract to be used between the THPF and the THPF participant. The contract shall include:

(a). The rights of each party; and

(b). Responsibilities of each party.

6. The procedures for determining the amount of allowance provided to each THPF participant, and the schedule for disbursement.

7. Procedures for payment or monitoring of utilities, telephone and rent.

8. Description of proposed THPF participant living unit furnishings and policy regarding disposition of furnishings when the THPF participant completes the program.

9. Procedures for evaluating the THPF participant's progress.

10. Procedures for the development, review implementation and modification of the needs and services plan for participants placed in the THPF.

11. The emergency plan that shall include emergency information, instructions and telephone numbers, including a 24-hour emergency number for the licensee and the participants' responsible party. The licensee shall ensure that each staff and resident understands and is capable of implementing the plan.

12. Administrator: All licensees shall have an administrator who meets one of the following requirements:

    a). A Master's Degree from an accredited graduate school on social work or social welfare, marriage, family and child counseling, counseling psychology or human services degree. In addition, the administrator shall have documented ability and leadership through a minimum of three years of experience in the field of child or family services, two years of which have been in an administrative or managerial position.

    (b). A Bachelor's Degree in a behavioral science from an accredited college or university. In addition, the administrator shall have demonstrated ability and leadership through a minimum of five years of experience in the field of child or family services, two years of which have been in an administrative or managerial position. The administrator shall be responsible for the operation of the THPF. The administrator shall be present in the THPF at least twenty hours per week during business hours. At all other times, when the administrator is absent from the THPF, there shall be coverage by the administrator's designee. If the designee does not meet the administrator qualifications there shall be immediate access to the administrator or one who meets the administrator requirements. The administrator's designee shall have knowledge of the THPF operations, training in programs provided by the THPF.

The THPF shall employ or retain qualified consultants necessary to implement the plan of operation.

V. What standards apply to long-term care facilities?

California's oversight of long-term care facilities is the most rigorous in the nation and the most comprehensive for any category of provider in the state. The Department of Health Services, the Department of Social Services, the Department of Mental Health and the Department of Developmental Services each play a role in licensing and regulating care providers.

Providers must meet state licensure standards, and in the skilled setting are also governed by a stringent set of federal requirements. In addition, several other federal, state and local agencies including the Federal Health Care Financing Administration, State Departments of Aging, Justice and Consumer Affairs and the Office of the State Fire Marshal also review facility services in California. Facilities must demonstrate compliance with hundreds of very detailed regulations. To ensure compliance with these standards, California state surveyors annually conduct thorough inspections of each facility.

VI. What is the role of the state in the welfare system?

State agencies play an important role in the management and general oversight of long-term care services. The state **Health & Human Services Agency** has primary responsibility over long-term care providers. The various Departments under Health & Human Services have specific responsibilities:

1. The **Department of Health Services** is responsible for licensing health facilities, home health agencies and hospices, and for general oversight of the services they provide.

2. The **Department of Social Services** manages California's integrated social service and income maintenance programs. The Department's Community Care Licensing Division licenses residential care facilities, and Adult and

Family Services Division is responsible for monitoring elder abuse.

3. The **Department of Developmental Services** is responsible for services to Californians with developmental disabilities such as mental retardation, cerebral palsy, epilepsy and autism.

4. The **Department of Mental Health** sets overall policy for the delivery of mental health services; establishes priorities, standards and procedures within which mental health services operate; assists in planning programs; monitors, reviews and evaluates the actual operation of services; and oversees any changes brought about by the evaluation and review process.

5. The **Department of Aging** serves as the focus for community-based services to California's seniors. Its mission is to provide leadership in addressing issues related to aging Californians, and in developing community-based systems of long-term care services throughout the state.

6. The **Ombudsman Program** advocates for the rights of all residents of 24-hour long-term care facilities and adult day health care centers in the state.

In addition to the Health & Human Services agencies, other state and local agencies, such as State and County Fire Marshals, Cal-OSHA, and the Department of Consumer Affairs also have roles in the oversight of long-term care in California. Nursing facilities are subject to an extensive set of standards prescribed in state licensing law and federal Medicare/Medicaid certification requirements. State inspectors spend hundreds of hours each year enforcing these regulations in their annual compliance visits to each of California's long-term care facilities.

Assisted living/Residential Care Facility for the Elderly (RCFE) providers are surveyed annually by the Dept. of Social Services. Other long-term care programs for the aged and disabled have varying degrees of oversight from state and local agencies. As the role of the other programs grow and develop, public concern and government oversight is also expanding. Although regulation and enforcement activities will always be necessary, California needs a less polarized, more collaborative approach to quality that focuses on prevention, quality improvement and results management.

VII. FACTS ABOUT LONG-TERM CARE

- There are approximately 1,400 licensed nursing facilities in California. These facilities care for more than 250,000 Californians each year.
- There are approximately 6,000 assisted living/residential care facilities in California.
- There are approximately 775 ICF/DD-H homes and approximately more than 300 ICF/DD-N homes 771 in California.
- There are approximately 44 intermediate care facilities in California.
- The average nursing facility costs range between $101 and $120 per day ($37,000 - $44,000 per year).
- Assisted living rates range from $1,000 to $3,000 per month, depending on such variables as building design and amenities.
- Two-thirds of California's nursing home residents rely on Medi-Cal to pay for their care in a nursing facility. The average Medi-Cal reimbursement rate is $115 per day.
- Almost 100 percent of clients who reside in homes for the developmentally disabled rely on Medi-Cal to pay for their care.
- Medi-Cal does not pay for assisted living. About 90 percent of assisted living services are paid for with private funds.
- The average length of stay in an assisted living facility is 3.3 years.
- Three out of four long-term care residents are women.
- Approximately 85 percent of long-term care residents in California are age 65 or older.
- On average, nursing facility residents require some level of assistance with 3 or more of the activities of daily living, which include bathing, dressing, transferring, toileting and eating. Assisted living residents need help with on average 1.6 activities of daily living.

- California is projected to be one of the fastest growing states in the nation in total population. In California, the elderly population (age 65+) is expected to grow more than twice as fast as the total population. The elderly age group will have an average increase of 112% during the period 1990-2020.

Chapter 2: GETTING STARTED IN THE BUSINESS

IT STARTS WITH A ....DREAM

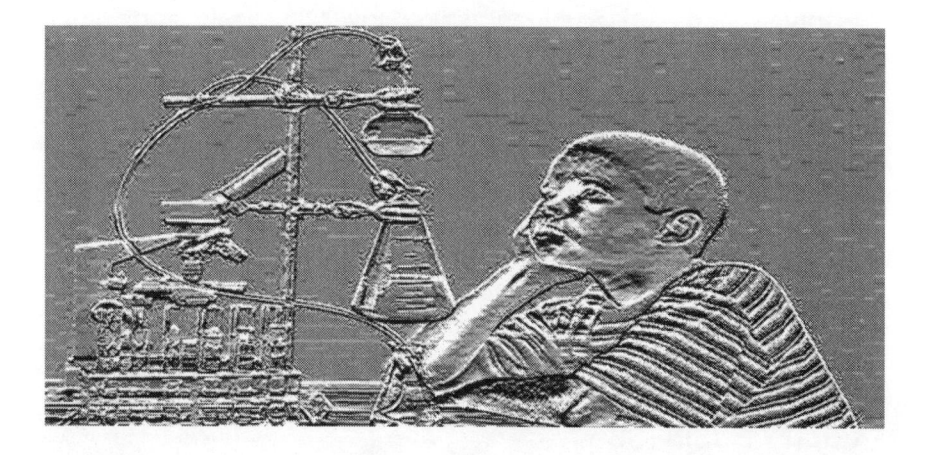

A. How to Steps in Setting up the Residential Care Facility Business

Create a Checklist

In order to get started, you need to have a general idea or a guideline to follow as to how the whole process works. Provided in this book are suggested steps that are enumerated in a form of a checklist that you might have to go through to be able to complete the whole process from start to finish. All the steps mentioned here are general guidelines only for purposes of establishing expectations. The steps may be interchangeable depending on particular situations that you will encounter, depending on the county or state agency regulations or requirements, steps may vary but the end results remain the same. It is important for you, the reader to be flexible and to observe the guidelines set forth by the local licensing regulation as well as that of the agency providing the business. For the sake of those who are new start-up individuals, these guidelines provided will definitely serve as a useful tool to follow.

First thing to do is to make a list of priority steps. These steps may vary depending on each and every individual situation in the application process. For instance, if you already have a business entity or existing property location for your facility, then you might have to move on to other steps that needed to be observed in order to be able to complete and submit your application for a license to operate a facility. Do not worry if you are unable to strictly observe the enumerated steps. As long as you cover the basic steps, your Licensing Program Analyst from Community Care Licensing will help you walk through it in form of consultation on revisions or addendum to your application. Also, remember that the process and steps observed in regards to responding to a **Request For a Proposal RFP** may be slightly different from what is stated in the standard application process. In responding to an RFP, worry not because this book also covers the subject briefly to give you a better idea on what you will expect in the RFP process.

"HOW TO" STEPS IN SETTING UP THE COMMUNITY CARE FACILITY BUSINESS

Step 1: Attend an 8-Hour Initial Orientation Class sponsored by your local Community Care Licensing office and try to secure the required Attendance Orientation Affidavit which will provide a window period of six (6) months to accomplish the required three (3) stages/components of the application process. **(First Stage/ Component of Affidavit)**

(Time line: 8 Hours)

Step 2: Become a Certified Facility Administrator.
(Time line: 30-90 days)

(a). Schedule yourself to attend an Initial Administrator Certification Course sponsored by a state recognized/vendorized private agency or school that provide the required initial certification classes. The required hours may vary 40 hours for Group Home and Residential Care Facility for the Elderly, and the Chronically Ill, and 35 Hours for Adult Residential Care Facility.

(b). Take the State Certification Exam and Pass it. Within sixty (60) days from date of completion of the certification class, the applicant must be able to pass the state exam.

(c). Get Fingerprinted by Live-Scan and secure background check clearance from FBI-DOJ.

(d). Secure CPR-First Aid Certification.

(e). For Adult/Senior Facilities, Administrator must attend and secure eight (8) hours HIV-Hepatitis certification.

(f). Direct Support Professionals: Direct support professionals in Service Levels 2, 3, and 4 facilities employed before January 1, 2001 must satisfactorily complete the first 35-hour training segment (Year1) by January 1, 2002; and satisfactorily complete the second 35-hour training segment (Year 2) by January 1, 2003. Direct support professionals in Service Levels 2, 3, and 4 facilities employed on or after January 1, 2001, have one year from date of hire to satisfactorily complete the first 35-hour training segment; and, two years from the date of hire to complete the second 35-hour training segment.

Direct care staff DCS/employees working in group homes for children with levels 1 to 14, must be able to complete 40 hours of continuing education units CEU's within two (2) from date of initial hire in order to maintain active employment status in the group home.

Step 3: Create a Business Plan   *(Time line: 30 to 90 days)*

Prepare a Start-Up Cost / Budget Cost

Financing the Business

Step 4: Prepare Draft of Program Design.
(Time line: 30-60 days)

Step 5: Establish your Entity: Corporation, Sole Proprietorship, Partnership, Limited Liability Corporation.
(Time line: 30-60 days)

- Register the business entity with the local county where business will be established like the Secretary of State, City Hall, etc..

- Secure Fictitious Business Name Statement

- Contact your local IRS, Franchise Tax Board, business license from City Hall, etc... Secure For Profit or Not for Profit Status through IRS-Franchise Tax Board.

- Open a business bank account.

- Advertise in the local newspaper for job applicants, secure staff, consultants ready for work upon license approval.

Step 6: Purchase vs. Leasing a Property/Business?

- Lease a property as the facility: An alternative choice.
(Time line: 30-60 days)

Step 7: Secure Host Letter. Furnish copy of program design to city council, city planning representatives and secure host letter from the county/ city where facility is established.
(Time line: 30-60 days)

Step 8: Get Your Business Facility Insured. *(Time line: 30 days)*

- General and Professional Liability Insurance to include abuse and allegation and other blanket insurances to protect yourself and your staff.

- Property and Transportation Coverage.

- Other related Insurance coverage (ask you local insurance broker)

Step 9: Submit Application Packet: License to Operate a Facility. **(Second Stage/Component)** Together a with the list of the different requirements specified for a given facility to the Community Care Licensing. (See three stages of the application process)
(Time line: 90 days)

An Easy Guide On How to Establish Your First Residential Care Facility

Step 10: Request for Fire Marshal Inspection of the Property
(Time line: 15-30 days)

Step 11: Secure Vendorization Packet: For Adults ARF, GH and Senior RCFE Facilities, in order to receive referral clients, it must be vendorized. The facility / applicant must schedule with the respective agency who is responsible for placing consumers to the facility such as Dept. of Children and Family Services, Child Protective Services, Adult Protective Services, Dept. of Aging, Regional Center, Dept. of Mental Health etc.. In some agencies, orientation process may take place for at least forty (40) hours.

(Time line: 30-60 days)

Placement agency representative to visit the applicant facility.

Final Review of Application: Ninety (90) Day Review from date of receipt of application.

Return application for revision, approval or denial. If correction is required, the applicant must respond within 30 days from date of notice of correction.

Second Visit from Community Care Facility representative and provide consultation on any more items missed during the first visit. (Optional)

Respond to a Request For Proposal (RFP) optional (In RFP, Steps 1-14 may be applicable but not in all instances)

Step 12: Community Care Licensing Representative to visit the facility to confirm compliance with the regulation

(Third Stage / Component)
(Time line: 60-90 days from date application is submitted)

Second visit from placement agencies (optional)

Orientation from Community Care Licensing and Regional Center or placing agencies.

Step 13: Secure Approval of License to Operate. Issuance of Provisional License (if no pending major issues on the application. *(Time line: 60-90 from date of application submission)*

Step 14: Business officially begins upon receipt of the provisional license to operate. Clients referred to the applicant facility.

Although the steps mentioned here may vary from state to state or from agency to another, these steps enumerated will give the reader/applicant a generalized expectation on the application process from initial stage up to initial operation of the business.

An Easy Guide On How to Establish Your First Residential Care Facility

Start to Finish: Projected Time Line

Month 1 Month 2 Month 3 Month 4 Month 5 Month 6 Month 7 Month 8

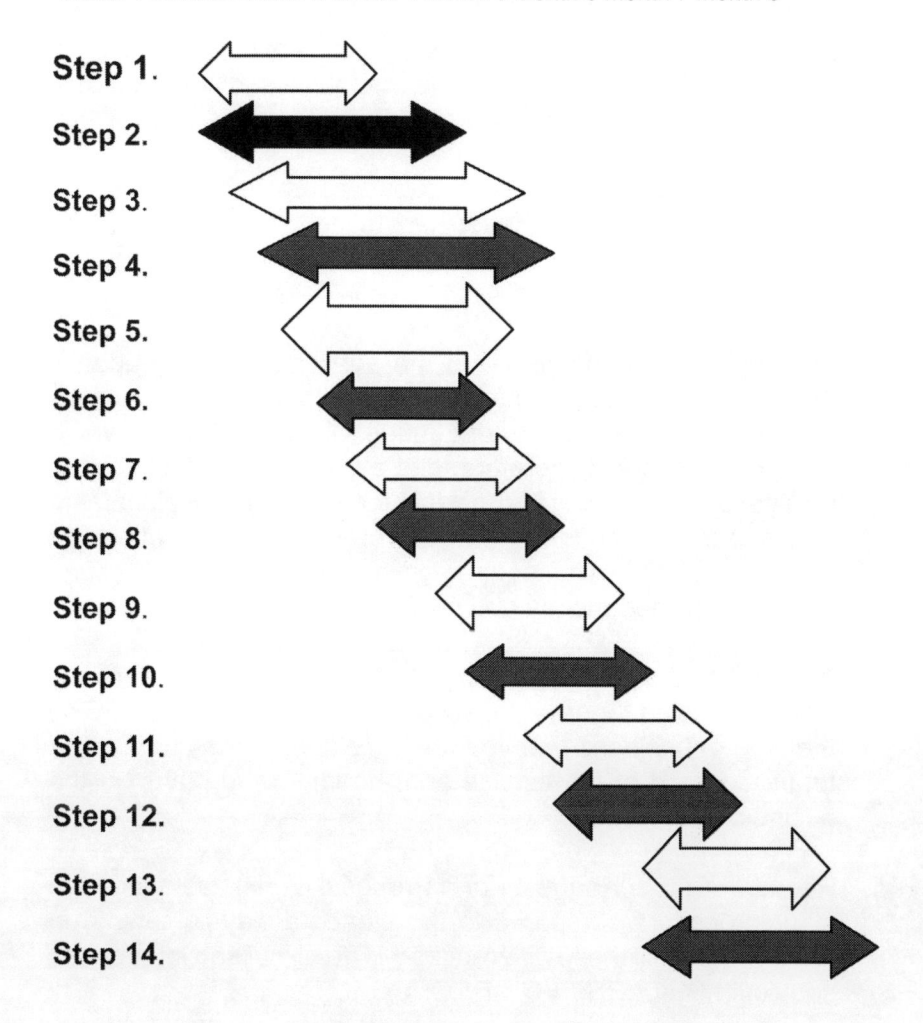

Step 1.

Step 2.

Step 3.

Step 4.

Step 5.

Step 6.

Step 7.

Step 8.

Step 9.

Step 10.

Step 11.

Step 12.

Step 13.

Step 14.

B. Things to consider when establishing the facility:

1. Facilities are categorized according to the level of care they provide which also corresponds to the amount of scheduled compensation to be received from the placement agencies, Medi-Cal, Dept. of Mental Health etc...

2. Receiving a license from Health Care Licensing and or Community Care Licensing to operate a facility does not automatically come with it the expectations of receiving clients/consumers to serve. Licensing is responsible for the issuance of a license to the facility, while placement agencies (Dept. of Social Services, Regional Center, Dept. of Aging etc..) are responsible for providing the clients/consumers to care for in these facilities. One must secure vendorization from the corresponding local placement agencies in order to receive clients/consumers to care for in the business.

3. The demand for the need on the services of every agency may depend on factors like location of facility, type of services provided by the home, current budget allocations and a whole lot of other factors. Therefore, it is a wise idea to first consult with the county agency responsible for the licensing, placement and resource allocation to find out where is a good location and for what type of facility requirements expected before investing your hard earned money and resources.

4. Attend the Initial Orientation sponsored by your local Community Care Licensing Agency to acquire important information on the type of business that you are considering, the current and future demand of the service and the long term plans on the business.

5. Responding to a Request For a Proposal (RFP) has a different steps/procedure compared to the standard way of setting up the business. All these differences will be discussed later on the subject of REQUEST FOR PROPOSAL.

An Easy Guide On How to Establish Your First Residential Care Facility

C. Checklist of important things to remember in keeping the facility operation within the required licensing standards.

Here are some of the important checklist of things that you need to observe when you conceptualize your future facility and explain in your own words how the following matters will be met and observed in your program design:

Cleanliness ☐

- The most important aspect of maintaining a good facility is that it must meet the standards of cleanliness and order. Explain how do you intend to observe it.

Patient Rights ☐

- There must be a written description of patient rights and responsibilities which copies must be furnished to the clients/consumers, social worker and families.
- Staff must protect patient privacy and dignity at all times.
- The use of restraints must be kept to a minimum.
- If restraints are used, it must be applied only after other alternatives have been exhausted.
- There must be a facility policy and procedure to uphold these rights.

Care Planning ☐

- Does it encourage family and agency involvement in the development of client's care plan, ISP, IPP needs and services plan, etc...
- In case of a restricted health there must be a plan to discuss, monitor and evaluate the needs of the clients.
- Will you provide services for the terminally ill residents and their families?
- Is your program able to accommodate consumers with disease including AIDS

Staff Attitudes ☐

- Will your staff show interest in, affection and respect for the residents?
- Observe courtesy at all times?
- Quick response to patient calls of assistance at all times?
- Provide a respectful and friendly environment
- Management's knowledge of available programs

Licensure and Certification ☐

- Administrator certificate and staff CEU's
- Is the facility certified to provide Medicare and/or Medi-Cal coverage if the individual needs it?
- Do you have the latest state survey available for review?
- Quality-assurance program

Location ☐

- Is the facility conveniently located for frequent visits and is accessible to family and friends?
- Is the facility located near a hospital?
- Is the facility conveniently located for the individual's physician(s)?

Costs ☐

- Charges within the standard

Medical ☐

- Physicians and health care professional availability in case of emergency.
- Are personal physicians allowed to treat individuals?
- Does the facility report to the individual's physician?
- Is regular medical attention guaranteed?
- Will your care plans and medical records be kept accordingly?
- Are individuals and families involved in treatment plans?
- How is confidentiality of medical record guaranteed?
- Is there a variety of medical services (dentists, podiatrists, optometrists) available for the residents?

- In an emergency, how will the individual's personal physician be notified?

Hospitalization ☐

- Does the facility have an arrangement with a nearby hospital?
- Will the facility provide emergency transportation?
- Are accommodations made to hold an resident's bed if that person is hospitalized?

Pharmacy ☐

- Do you have routine and emergency drugs locked at the facility?
- Does a pharmacist review individual drug treatment plans?
- Is a pharmacist available for individuals and staff?

Therapy Program ☐

- Is a physical therapy program available under the supervision of a qualified physical therapist?
- Are speech therapy and occupational therapy available?

Activities Program ☐

- Are individual preferences observed?
- Are group and individual activities available?
- Is participation encouraged?
- Are the individuals involved in their surrounding community?
- Does the facility have volunteers working with the residents?
- Are offsite trips planned?

Social Services ☐

- Is a social worker available to assist individuals and families?

Accident Prevention ☐

- Will the facility be kept clean and well lit?
- Will the facility be kept free of clutter and hazards?
- Will the furniture at the facility be appropriate?

- Will there be warning signs posted on freshly waxed or wet floors?
- Will you install handrails and grab bars in the hallways and bathrooms?

Fire Safety

- Is the facility compliant with state and federal codes?
- Are exits unobstructed and clearly marked?
- Are emergency evacuation plans posted with floor plans throughout the facility?
- How often will your facility staff conduct fire-disaster drills?
- Are exits unlocked from the inside?
- Are doors to stairways kept closed?

Bedrooms

- Do the bedrooms open onto the hallway?
- Does each of the resident rooms have a window?
- Are bedrooms limited to two beds?

Bedrooms

- Do the bedrooms open onto the hallway?
- Does each of the resident rooms have a window?
- Are bedrooms limited to two beds?
- Is each bed equipped with a nurse call bell?
- Will the bedrooms have night stand and chairs for each resident?
- Is each individual provided a separate clothes closet or set of drawers?
- Are the bedrooms wide and wheelchair-accessible?
- Is care a qualification used in roommate selection?
- Is each bed easily accessible?
- Are residents encouraged to decorate rooms with personal items?

Lobby

- Does it have welcoming atmosphere?
- Is the furniture attractive and comfortable?

- Is the activities schedule posted on a bulletin board?
- Are the facility certificates and licenses on display?

Hallways ☐

- Are the halls wide enough for two wheelchairs to pass easily?
- Are the halls well lit?

Dining Room ☐

- Is the dining area clean, attractive and inviting?
- Are tables convenient for wheelchairs?
- Is food tasty and appealing to the eye?
- Is there adequate time to eat meals?
- Do the meals match the posted menu?
- Is help given to the residents who need it?

Kitchen ☐

- Is the food preparation area separated from the dishwashing and garbage areas?
- Is food requiring refrigeration properly stored?
- Do the kitchen workers observe sanitation rules?

Food ☐

- Does a dietitian plan menus for residents requiring special diets?
- Are personal likes and dislikes considered?
- Does the menu vary from meal to meal?
- Is there adequate time to eat each meal?
- Does the facility provide snacks?
- Is food delivered to individuals unable to eat in the dining room?
- Are warm meals served warm?

Activity Rooms ☐

- Is there a designated area available for resident activities?
- Does the facility provide activity equipment, such as games, easels, yarn or a kiln?

- Is the equipment being used by residents?

Special Purpose Room ☐

- Are rooms set aside for therapy or physical examinations?
- Are rooms available for private visits with family and friends?

Isolation Room ☐

- Does the facility provide at least one bed and bathroom for patients with contagious illness?

Toilet Facilities ☐

- Are toilets convenient to bedrooms?
- Are they wheelchair accessible?
- Are nurse call bells located near each toilet?
- Are hand grips installed near each toilet?
- Are bathtubs and showers equipped with non-slip

Grounds ☐

- Are the grounds accessible to handicapped individuals?
- Does the facility provide outdoor furniture for residents and visitors?
- Is parking adequate for visitors?

Religious Observances ☐

- Does the facility make arrangements for patients to worship as they please?
- Is help given to the residents who need it?

Grooming ☐

- Is assistance available for bathing and grooming?
- Are barbers or beauticians available?
- Does the facility provide basic laundry service?

D. Types of Consumers/Clients Placed in Residential Care Facilities

In general, children placed in **Small Family Homes (SFH), Foster Family Homes (FFH), Foster Family Agency (FFA), Transitional Housing (TH), Group Homes (GH)** are those from displaced families as a result of abuse, neglect, inability to care for self due to disability, death of careprovider and for other reasons that the court/guardian deems necessary to protect the rights and interest of the children. For the purpose of protecting the children, cases are filed in court on their behalf and as a result of such pending case, children are placed either with relatives and friends and in some situations in these residential care homes on a temporary basis until the court makes final determination of whether they may come back home to their parents, relatives or a guardian or a court appointed representative or continue to stay in these placements until they turn 18 or eventually when ready to live a life they choose as an adult. Children placed in these homes may be categorized into two types:

(a) **"The High Risk Consumers"** those who are noted to be physically aggressive, emotionally disturbed and are most likely to become a threat to themselves and or to others, these children are placed in homes deemed according to Levels 1-14 which starts from the lowest type of care and supervision to the highest care which most definitely requires a more restricted environment.

Dependent Children

They are generally dependents of the Juvenile Court System and placed by county social services department. These children are mostly physically, sexually or emotionally abused, neglected or exploited or at risk of being abused neglected or exploited. They often have behavioral and/or emotional problems that prevent them from being cared for in a family type environment.

Juvenile Wards

Children who are juvenile offenders. These children are generally wards of the Juvenile Court and placed by county probation departments.

Seriously Emotionally Disturbed

Children who are identified as Seriously Emotionally Disturbed (SED) and require out-of-home placement in order to benefit from an educational program. These children are generally placed by county mental health agencies.

To have a better idea as to what type of clients/consumers you would like to care and supervise, you are encouraged to discuss with a licensing program analyst/coordinator from the county social services or probation department or other placing agencies to discuss the types of services that the department or placement agencies require to meet their needs. The analyst will present the types of services that meets the needs of the children under the juvenile justice system as well as the adults and seniors under the welfare system.

(b). **"The At-Risk Clients"** who by birth or other reasons acquired their medical, physical, mental or developmental disability which require them to benefit from receiving care from others and without such personalized care, they will be at risk of not surviving. These "at risk" consumers are considered as Developmentally Disabled. This also include children and adults who are limited by their physical disability and whose parents or person responsible for their well being can not take care of them due to financial or personal reasons. These children are generally placed by regional centers in a residential care setting if not in an institutional type of setting. These individuals are placed in homes with service levels between 1 to 4 depending on the degree of care and assistance they are expected to receive due partly to their disability. The disabilities are qualified as: Mental Retardation, Autism, Cerebral Palsy, Epilepsy and other forms of disabilities that causes or leads to mental retardation which an individual acquires by birth or prior to age 18, an individual is entitled to receive support from the state as mandated under the Lanterman-Petris-Short Act or simply Lanterman Act established in the mid 1970's. Children, adults and seniors living in these facilities are entitled to receive continued support sometimes for a lifetime or as long as they need it. **Upon reaching adult age and still in need of assistance**, they possibly will transition to live in an **Adult Residential Care Facility (ARF)** within levels 1 to 4. If and when they develop serious illness related to their disabilities, they may be recommended (if it is for their benefit) to live in an environment that require higher level of care, and such needs are provided for in an ICF-DDH, ICF-DD-N where these facilities provide a home-like setting with medical and health care professionals on board as staff to monitor their medical needs in a residential care setting.

As these adults turn seniors and remain to be unable to care for themselves, they shall be placed in Residential Care Facility for the Elderly (RCFE), perhaps for the rest of their lives should their mental and physical conditions continue to decline. While living in these types of residential care homes, the residents typically go to activity centers for their leisure and recreation. These centers are called **Adult or Senior Day Care Centers** and if they have medical issues that would restrict them from their normal routine, they could be participating in **Adult or Senior Day Health Care Centers**.

Should the health condition of these adults or seniors continue to decline further than medically necessary, as they become mentally, physically and/or medically fragile, they may be required to live in a more restricted environment where their health conditions are monitored constantly as they are susceptible to developing illnesses related or unrelated to their disabilities, then they may be required to be placed in a **Residential Care Facility for the Chronically Ill (RCFCI)**. This type of facility also accommodates individuals with other illnesses such as AIDS-HIV.

E. **Levels of care is equivalent to the level of pay for the services provided.**

The general premise is that the more difficult it is to care for the consumer as far as their needs and services are concerned, the more individualized the services that you as care-provider will provide. It also follows that the cost of the care services likewise increases. The higher the cost of services, the higher the pay scale that you will expect to receive on a monthly basis. Is that pretty confusing? Do not worry because I assure you that by the time you finish this chapter, you will have a better idea on what I am talking about.

Remember:

HIGH RISK CONSUMERS: (Group Home Children): LEVELS 1-14

AT RISK CONSUMERS (Developmentally Disabled Children, Adults and Seniors): LEVELS: 1-4

Now, let us review. If you are looking at serving consumers belonging to the High Risk Category, meaning children living in a Group Home setting, you are possibly considering levels 1 through 14 for your facility. If you are considering serving the developmentally disabled population, you are possibly considering service levels from 1 through 4 whether they are children, adults or seniors.

Now, you might ask: How do you know when the consumers you are serving belong to homes with Levels 1, 2, 4, 6, 10 up to 14 or from DD Levels 1 up to 4 ?

You need to remember this important information: Funds in residential care setting are coming from possibly two different funding resources also known as the referral placement agencies namely: (1). Dept. of Social Services paid for under the Foster Care Rates Bureau that oversees children placed in Group Homes, etc.. (2). Department of Aging, Dept. of Mental Health and 21 Regional Centers that places children, adults and seniors with developmental disabilities paid for through social services, welfare system, Medi-Cal, Medicaire, Medic-aide programs etc...

Note: *Residential care facilities must not combine in one placement both at risk and high risk clients as one will be a possible victim of the other.*

What is the significance of the LEVELS and what makes a certain facility qualify for a given level?

It is important at this learning stage to remember that LEVELS mentioned in this book ONLY refer to the level of care provided in the residential care facilities and not referring to the level of the clients or consumers YOU SERVE in the facility. The consumers are not considered according to their levels of disabilities because levels only refer particularly to the facilities and not the consumers. Consumers do not have levels and can not be categorized. Please be very sensitive about this matter. Service levels are differentiated by the amount of "direct supervision and specialized services" provided for the consumers in the facilities. Specialized services refer to the training, treatment and or supervision required in the care of the client/consumer as reflected in their service objectives at home and at the day program known as IPP/ISP.

All care providers including its administrative and direct care staff must undergo a 70-Hour Competency Based Training and Testing administered by the county regional occupational program ROP. This standardized training program is focused on meeting the increasing need for a higher level of care in residential care setting. As observed in most studies conducted, home care setting is more favorable than the institution setting. Therefore, the vision of integrating everyone into the community is no longer a remote possibility as you will eventually see a gradual increase in the establishment of quality residential care homes within the next few years. With this in mind, the private and the public agencies are now left with the responsibility of improving their quality of care services in these types of homes or face the consequence of probable extinction.

The levels reflect the following factors:

(a). Types of services

(b). Number of Hours and staffing ratio reflected on the services.

(c). Education, experiences and specialized training of its providers, administrator and staff.

(d). Qualifications and standards of quality care setting.

Levels referred to these homes signify the cost of providing and maintaining the services. In the succeeding page you will find a reference chart indicating the levels of care together with their corresponding pay rate for the services to be rendered. However, the figures represented may not be accurate because each level of services and their corresponding cost may vary for multitude of practical reasons such as county to county, state to state, agency to agency regulations as well as the state and federal budget allocations for these programs. In order to give you a broad idea on the explanation of the levels mentioned earlier and the presentation of corresponding amount on given levels, the reader will have a better understanding of the explanation behind the levels of care services.

First, you need to understand the different standards that qualify a home to be granted level from 1 to 14 and later identify the qualifications for a facility under levels 1 to 4. In general, remember that the amount of compensation for a given service corresponds appropriately to the amount and type of services provided for the consumer. The general qualification of a service level depends on factors such as the number of staff and professional services provided as part of the service, the types of daily and regular activities, level of care, therapy, counseling, supervision, and other services deemed to benefit the consumers in the facility. In short, the amount of compensation that one is expected to receive is always relative to the corresponding amount of services and effort rendered. This book does not attempt to explain every applicable law and regulation and does not guarantee the accuracy of the information as well as the figures presented. For more information, it is best to contact your local community care licensing office in your area.

LEVELS 1 TO 14   (Applies to Group Homes For High Risk Children)

For levels 1 to 14, these levels are known mainly in the group home setting as Rate Classification Level RCL. These are rate level categories for a group home program based on the care and services provided for in residential care homes. Each service level corresponds to a standardized rate of pay for the corresponding services provided. When the applicant for a group home license submits an application to the local community care licensing office, one of the things to be stated in the application is the group home program Rate Classification Level (RCL) which signifies a promise by the facility operator to provide designated services to the children in the placement. Each RCL correspond to a given number of hours and the quality of services provided which in turn are converted into accumulated points relative to the number of paid awake hours worked by qualified staff in three components namely: Child Care and Supervision, Social Work, and Mental Health Treatment Services.

If at the end of the fiscal year from initial date of operation, the facility failed to provide the quality of services as stated on the condition for a license, the facility will be subjected to an audit and an overpayment action may be imposed or collected. These deficiency payments shall be paid to the Department of Social Services or the agency that provided the funding for the services. In the succeeding year(s), if the facility continues to receive the RCL payments but provide inadequate services to the consumers by performing below the required RCL standard specified in the license, and the facility fails to maintain the minimum cumulative points for the given RCL, it is suggested that the facility should request for an adjustment of RCL by submitting a Program Rate Change Application to the Foster Care Rates Bureau to make the necessary adjustments in rate payments.

Hiring workers who meet higher education and experience requirements may increase monthly points associated with your RCL. The board of directors should ensure that the administrator takes steps to verify the level of education, experience, training and monthly paid awake hours of childcare workers, social workers, and mental health professionals, and compliant with fingerprint and Child Abuse Index requirements.

In the case of the Adult Residential Care Facility (ARF) and the Residential Care Facility for the Elder (RCFE) and the Chronically Ill (RCFCI) pay scale is based on levels 1 through 4 which in relation to the principle that the pay scale is based on the number of hours of services provided on a regular basis. This means that the more services the home provides, the more staff is on the payroll. The more staff that provides the therapy and personal services, the more costly it could get. The amount of the pay schedule varies from county to another and from one year to the other, therefore, it is better for the reader to inquire from the orientation participants/host or the placement agencies with regard to the amount of pay they are expecting to establish for their business as rates vary.

For those who are interested in becoming foster parents, foster families are the second choice of placement after relative resources are exhausted and before a child is placed in a residential care setting for obvious reasons and one of them is that, if the court system can not find family members to care for these children, foster families come in as second choice. If the child needs a more restricted type of environment due to behavior, mental health or medical issues, then a group home on the first five levels is the next choice. Should the type of care require a higher level, the placing agency may opt to secure services from succeeding levels in the facility setting until the appropriate needs and services are met accordingly. In this section, you will find sample standard rates normally paid for services in residential care facilities.

LEVEL 1 TO 4 (APPLIES TO FACILITIES FOR AT RISK CHILDREN, ADULTS AND SENIORS WITH DEVELOPMENTAL DISABILITY)

Let us all be reminded that the level for homes that accommodates children and adults with developmental disabilities such as the Group Homes, ARF's, including seniors living in RCFE are determined in a manner similar but not identical to how level 1 to 14 qualifications are made. Principles of qualification may be similar in nature but not necessarily identical in a sense that Levels 1 to 14 are standards set by Foster Care Rates Bureau FCRB while Levels 1 to 4 are standards set by Medi-Cal and placement agencies. Should the quality of care service is greater, so is the amount of the cost.

Level Types:

If clients are children in a Group Home setting are of the high risk category, then homes will be presumed within the **Levels 1 to 14**.

An Easy Guide On How to Establish Your First Residential Care Facility

If clients in a Group Home setting are developmentally disabled, mentally ill or medically fragile, the homes will be presumed to be within the **Levels 1 to 4** simply because services are paid through Medi-Cal and Regional Center system. In the case of day program or senior centers, clients/consumers are accommodated according to the center's ability to meet their needs. In day programs or adult/senior centers, levels do not apply because day programs are designed to accommodate clients/consumers based on their particular needs and service requirements. In general, consumers who do not require the use of specialized medical equipment such as oxygen tank, baclofen pump etc..., almost everyone with developmental disabilities with lower functioning capacities participate in center based day programming activities. For the consumers/clients with higher functioning potentials, they participate in community based programming activities and oftentimes transition to attend adult vocational schools or even colleges and universities. For consumers who by their fragile condition but are not confined in their beds, yet may require medical support of a Registered Nurse, they may be accommodated in an adult or senior day health care centers where programming activities may be limited to qualified functional skills development.

In order to better understand Levels 1 through 4, please refer to a sample table in this book which illustrates the different levels. The format illustrated here intends to simplify your understanding of what Level 1-14 is in relation to Level 1-4. In actual practice, this illustration may not be sharply accurate because of reasons mentioned earlier in this chapter.

Group Home Levels 1 thru 14			
Group Homes Levels:	**Level 1-4**	**Level 5-8**	**Level 9-11**	**Level 12-14**
Operation:				
Staff Operated	Yes	Yes	Yes	Yes
Owner Operated	Yes/No	No	No	No
Programming:				
Constant Supervision	Yes	Yes	Yes	Yes
Self-Dependency	Yes	Yes	No	No
Assaultive	No	No/Yes	Yes	Yes
Fire setting	No	No	No/Yes	Yes
Destructive	No	No	No/Yes	Yes
AWOL Risk	No	No	Yes	Yes
Gang Affiliation	No	No	No/Yes	Yes
Drugs	No	No	No/Yes	Yes
Violent Behavior	No	No	No	Yes
Academic Def.	Yes	Yes	Yes	Yes
Threat to others and to self	No	No	No/Yes	Yes
Self-Inflicted Behavior	No	No/Yes	Yes	Yes
Seizures	Yes	Yes	Yes	Yes
Behavior Deficits	No	No	Yes	Yes
Self-help needs	No	Yes	Yes	Yes
Self-feeding Assist	No	Yes/No	Yes	Yes
Medical Issues	No	No	No	Yes

An Easy Guide On How to Establish Your First Residential Care Facility

Group Homes Levels:	Level 1-4	Level 5-8	Level 9-11	Level 12-14
Mobility Assist	No	No/Yes	Yes	Yes
Staffing Ratio To Client	1:4 or 1:6	1:4	1:3	1:3 1:2 or 1:1
Qualifications of Staff experience	6 mos to 1 year	1 year	1 to 2 Years	2 to 3 years
Administrator Experience	6 mos to 1 year	1 year	1 to 2 years	2 to 3 years
Therapists	No	No	Yes	Yes
Social Worker	No	Yes	Yes	Yes
In-House RN	No	No	Yes	Yes
In-House Physician	No	Yes	Yes	Yes
Psychologist	No	Yes	Yes	Yes
Psychiatrist	No	Yes	Yes	Yes
Rec. Therapist	No	Yes	Yes	Yes
Physical Therapist	No	Yes	Yes	Yes
Behaviorist	No	Yes	Yes	Yes
Occ. Therapist	No	Yes	Yes	Yes
Facility Manager	Yes	Yes	Yes	Yes
Speech Therapist	Yes	Yes	Yes	Yes
Nutritionist	No	Yes	Yes	Yes
Additional Staff	No	No/Yes	Yes	Yes

Residential Care Facility for Developmentally Disabled Children, Adults and Seniors

Levels: ARF, GH RCFE, RCFCI	Level 1	Level 2	Level 3	Level 4
Operation:				
Staff Operated	Yes	Yes/No	Yes	Yes
Owner Operated	Yes	Yes/No	No	No
Programming:				
Constant Supervision	Yes	Yes	Yes	Yes
Self-Dependency	Yes	Yes	No	No
Assistance	Yes	Yes	Yes	Yes
Feeding	No	No/Yes	Yes	Yes
Dressing	No	No/Yes	Yes	Yes
Toileting	No	No/Yes	Yes	Yes
Transferring	No	No/Yes	Yes	Yes
Medication	No	No/Yes	Yes	Yes
Hygiene	No	No/Yes	Yes	Yes
Money Mgt	Yes	Yes	Yes	Yes/No
Medical Issues	No	No/Yes	Yes	Yes
Threat to others and to self	No	No	No/Yes	Yes
Self-Inflicted Behavior	No	Yes	Yes	Yes
Seizures	Yes	Yes	Yes	Yes
Behavior Issues	No	Yes	Yes	Yes
AWOL Risk	No	No	Yes	Yes

An Easy Guide On How to Establish Your First Residential Care Facility

Levels: ARF, GH RCFE, RCFCI	Level 1	Level 2	Level 3	Level 4
Behavior deficits	No	Yes	Yes	Yes
Self-help needs	No	Yes	Yes	Yes
Self-feeding Assist	No	No/Yes	Yes	Yes
Aggressive Beh	No	Yes	Yes	Yes
Destructive Behavior	No	Yes	Yes	Yes
Mobility Assist	No	No/Yes	Yes	Yes
Aggressive Behavior	No	No	Yes	Yes
Staffing ratio	1 staff to 4/6	1 staff to 4	1 staff to 3	1 staff to 3/2/1
Qualifications of Staff experience	6 mos to 1 year	1 year	1 to 2 Years	2 to 3 years
Administrator Experience	6 mos to 1 year	1 year	1 to 2 years	2 to 3 years
Therapists	Yes	Yes	Yes	Yes
Social Worker	No	Yes	Yes	Yes
In-House RN	No	No	Yes	Yes
In-House Dr.	No	Yes	Yes	Yes
Psychologist	No	No/Yes	Yes	Yes
Psychiatrist	No	No/Yes	Yes	Yes
Rec. Therapist	No	No/Yes	Yes	Yes
Physical Therapist	No	Yes	Yes	Yes
Behaviorist	No/Yes	Yes	Yes	Yes
Occ. Therapist	No/Yes	No/Yes	Yes	Yes

Levels: ARF, GH RCFE, RCFCI	Level 1	Level 2	Level 3	Level 4
Facility Manager	Yes	Yes	Yes	Yes
Speech Therapist	Yes	Yes	Yes	Yes
Nutritionist	Yes	Yes	Yes	Yes
Additional Staff	No	No/Yes	Yes	Yes

Who Pays For What?

Type of Facility	Medi-Cal	Placement Agency
Group Home / Foster Homes / FFA	Yes Medi-Caland FCRB	CPS/DCFS AFDC
Adult Residential Care	Yes	Regional Centers
Adult Day Care Center	Yes	Regional Centers
Adult Day Health Care	Yes	Regional Centers
Residential Care Facility for the Elderly	Yes/ +	Regional Centers / Dept. of Aging
Residential Care for the Chronically ILL	Yes/ +	Regional Centers/ Dept. of Aging
Senior Day Care Center	Yes/ +	Regional Centers/ Dept. of Aging
Senior Health Care Center	Yes/ +	Regional Centers/ Dept. of Aging

F. How do you get paid for the services provided in the facility and who pays for the long-term care services?

Between 1990 and year 2020, there will be approximately 87 Million Americans who will turn 65 and over and they will be in need of some form of personal care either in a residential care setting or in private homes. As America ages, there is an urgent need to address this growing problem and the question on who will pay for the health care cost remains in the balance. A recent study indicates that one in five Americans age 50 or over may need long-term care sometime within the next 12 months.

Although Medicare reform is a national priority, it can not help the vast majority of Americans who require facility-based long-term care. Medicare coverage of nursing facility care is very limited only covering the first 20 days of care in most cases.

a). Medicaid (known as Medi-Cal in California)

Nearly two-thirds of all who live in nursing care facilities and residential care homes rely on Medi-Cal. The proportion is even higher at facilities caring for people with developmental disabilities, where nearly 100 percent of clients are Medi-Cal beneficiaries. This means that a big portion of what Medi-Cal funding pays for medications, hospitalizations including care homes. Unfortunately, seniors must deplete their life savings and impoverish themselves in order to become eligible for Medicaid. The objective of the Medicaid program is to provide essential medical care and services to preserve the health by alleviating sickness and mitigate handicapping conditions for individuals or families receiving public assistance, or those whose income is not sufficient to meet their individual needs. The paid or covered services include standard medical services required in the treatment or prevention of diseases, disability, infirmity or impairment. Every state in the nation designs its own programs within broad federal guidelines. Thus, Medicaid programs vary from state to state.

b). Medicare.

Medicare is administered by the U.S. Department of Health and Human Services (HHS), a federal insurance program for people age 65 and over, disabled for at least two years; or suffering from chronic kidney disease. Nursing facility coverage under Medicare is very limited. The average length of stay paid for by Medicare is 26 days. Nationally, only about 4 percent of nursing facility patient days are supported by Medicare. California slightly exceeds this national statistic, having approximately 8% percent of its long-term care population supported by Medicare.

c). Long Term Care Insurance

Long-term care insurance can protect an individual's assets and provide peace of mind. A good long-term care insurance policy will cover all levels of care, especially personal care, and all settings, including facility care, community adult day care, assisted living facilities and nursing facilities.

The cost of a long-term care insurance policy primarily depends on the age of the policyholder when purchased. The annual premium for a low-option policy for a person at age 50 is about $400. This same policy for a 65-year-old person is about $1,100 per year; for a person age 79, the policy would cost more than $4,300. Recognizing the growing need for better insurance coverage, the State of California formed the Partnership for Long-Term Care, an innovative program offered by the Department of Health Services in cooperation with a select number of private insurance companies. The insurance companies who participate in the program have agreed to offer high quality policies that meet stringent requirements set by the Partnership and the State of California. For more information, call toll-free (800) 434-0222.

d). Supplemental Security Income/State Supplementary Programs (SSI/SSP)

SSI is a federal cash benefit program for those over 65 years of age, the blind and the disabled. SSI is the only government source of payment for RCFE/assisted living residents, as Medi-Cal does not pay for the RCFE setting. SSI is supplemented by the State of California to assist in paying for RCFE services. The SSI grant may provide the total monthly income or it may supplement a low income. In California, approximately 30 percent of the RCFE residents are recipients of SSI.

e). Third Party Payors

This category of financing includes individual insurance plans other than Medicare or Medi-Cal; Veteran's Benefits; Municipal Assistance benefits; and long term care insurance policies. These sources account for about 9 percent of long term care payment.

For the purpose of limiting our discussion on the coverage for the different types of residential care setting applicable to the business we will be focusing on group home and residential care facilities for adults and seniors. The topic on payment for services provided in these types of facilities will be a bit confusing from the start but as you go along with the reading, you will eventually understand the basic information that you need to know. In order to have a clearer understanding of how the facility is paid for the services provided, the matter is elaborated briefly based on two categories of consumers to service namely: a). The High Risk Consumers and the 2). At Risk Consumers.

For a better understanding of how to receive payments for services, one will need to know more about benefits being received from Medi-Cal. Information about Medi-Cal benefits may be acquired by calling the local public agency or Social Security office and ask for literature on benefits. Later on in the business, you will eventually get to know more specifics on Medi-Cal, but just for the sake of understanding the basics on Medi-Cal, the general rule is that: people who are in the system by qualifications such as disability, illness, age or minor children under protective custody of the state are entitled to receive benefits from Medi-Cal. Medi-Cal most of the times pay for the board and care (housing and lodging), programming (activities at the home or facility), medications, food, specialized equipment, therapy, etc.... and other expenses deemed necessary by the public agency that places these individuals. Since there are varied categories of facilities mentioned in this book, explore the answer to the question of how payments are received and paid by understanding how the different types of facilities function. Remember, each facility except group homes for CPS/DCFS children is paid from different county/state programs and to name the most common sources are **Medi-Cal, Medi-Care and Medic-Aide, and at times the placement agencies such as Regional Centers which supports the expenses such as cost of living in a board and care facilities, programming expenses etc...**

which play a very important role in most if not all of these residential care program expenses.

To mention just a few of the services paid thru Medi-Cal, room and board, daily programming activities, medications, consultation visits, dental, physical, psychological, therapeutic, hospitalizations, special medical equipment and accessories and adaptive equipment, and for most adult and seniors; it also pays for the placements in hospitals, residential care facilities such as the homes enumerated unless the placement agency such as Dept. of Aging, Regional Centers etc... for special arrangements or medical reasons pays for their share of cost of living in facilities including hospitalization sometimes when Medi-Cal is unable to cover the difference.

For the first five categories of residential care facilities such as homes that care and supervise children particularly those living in Small Family Home, Foster Family Home, Group Home and Transition Home, the company that wishes to serve these categories are paid from the funds allocated for the Aid to Families with Dependent Children-Foster Care (AFDC-FC) whereby these funds generally pay the costs for children who are placed by county social services or probation departments. The AFDC-FC funding comes from combined resources of State/County or Federal dollars. The AFDC-FC funds are paid to the children's home care providers for the services given provided that the following conditions are met:

1. The facility/group home program must have the written support of the host county, the primary placing county or regional consortium of counties. The county where the group home/facility will be located shall serve as the "host county ".

2. The facility/group home must be licensed by the Community Care Licensing Division (CCLD).

3. The group home must be organized and operated on a non-profit basis (as indicated and verified by a Federal IRS tax exemption letter or a copy of the articles of incorporation filed by the group home corporation with the California Secretary of State).

4. The group home "program" must have an AFDC-FC rate established by the California Department of Social Services (CDSS) Foster Care Rates Bureau (FCRB). A group home "program" shall contain a unique combination of services that will be provided to specific types of children in one or more licensed group homes. The group home will receive payments according to the services that the facility intended to provide. The FCRB will determine the rates/fees (Rate Classification Level RCL) based on a standard format of computation that is provided which will serve as a basis for the corresponding services rendered to the clients/children.

For those group homes that will care for children who are developmentally disabled and are referred by the Regional Centers, they shall be paid through Medi-Cal, Medicare and Medic-aide and at times when special programming is required, Regional Center pays for the share of cost. However, there are also some developmentally disabled children who may be eligible for the AFDC-FC Funding.

Children placed by private individuals, institutions or other agencies including county mental health agency, may have their own resources to cover the costs of the placement.

How much do you get paid for the services?

For the purpose of giving the reader a general idea as to how much facilities are paid for their services, included in this section, are two sample pay scales for the categories discussed earlier. If the date of printing of this material render the figures obsolete, it is advisable for the reader to make the necessary adjustments for their own purpose. The reader might find the projected figures very useful in writing a business plan or in establishing decision as to whether the undertaking is worth a try.

Medi-Cal pays for the board and care expenses including food and lodging, clothing and basic needs at a standard rate. The placement agency such as Regional Center or other agencies, (if Medi-Cal does not cover and the service is necessary) pays for the programming cost at the facility such as services provided for the consumer's in form of therapy, activities, day program, etc... Medical and dental needs including other health care related services are paid by Denti-Cal and Medi-Cal. The rate schedule only applies to homes and facilities that serve the needs of the developmentally disabled individuals. However, in the case of high risk children living in foster homes and group homes including specialized homes, the rate schedule may be different as the fund resources come from the Dept. of Social Services Foster Care Rates Bureau. The types of levels in these types of home for children are categorized accordingly from level 1 thru 14, one being the lowest in restriction and gradually increasing in level of supervision and care depending on the types of services provided for the children. On the first six levels, the home may be operated either by the owner of the facility or a staff or both. As the level increases from level six and above, so is the type of level of care and supervision which owner-operated facilities may find it practical to be staff operated instead due to the increase in stress and job requirements.

ALTERNATIVE RESIDENTIAL MODEL RATES (Effective 01-01-04) through (12-31-04) Residential Care Facilities for the Developmentally Disabled.

The sample rate chart courtesy of Inland Regional Center indicating effective date as 01-01-04 up to 12-31-04 which means that rates may be inaccurate as they vary with factors such as time of printing, area coverage, county and agency involved etc... (These rates may be inaccurate so reader is advised to research or contact his/her local licensing agency for more information. Tip: Estimate to add at least 10% per year as margin of increase).

(Chart / Rates courtesy of Community Care Licensing and Regional Center January 2004)

An Easy Guide On How to Establish Your First Residential Care Facility

Board and Care Rates and Classification Levels

Level 1	Board and Care	$ 853.00 ($ 28.02/ day)	$ 853.00 ($ 28.02/ day)	Owner OR /Staff Operated: **$ 853/Mo**
Level 2	Board and Care	$ 853.00 ($ 28.02/ day)	$ 853.00 ($ 28.02/ day)	
Plus	Regional Center Costs	$ 841.00 ($ 27.63/ day)	$ 1,051 ($ 34.53/ day)	Owner Oper: **$ 1,694/Mo** Staff Oper: **$ 1,904/Mo**
Level 3	Board and Care	$ 853.00 ($ 28.02/ day)	$ 853.00 ($ 28.02/ day)	
Plus	Regional Center Costs	$ 1,095.00 ($ 35.97/ day)	$ 1,367.00 ($ 44.91/ day)	Owner Oper: **$ 1,948/Mo** Staff Oper: **$ 2,220/Mo**
Level 4 Plus	Board and Care	**All level 4s are staff operated**	**Basic rate: $ 853.00** ($ 28.02/ day)	
A	Regional Center Costs	Basic Rate +	$ 2,002 ($ 65.77/ day)	**$2,855.00/ Mo.**
B	Regional Center Costs	Basic Rate +	$ 2,190.00 ($ 71.95/ day)	**$ 3,043.00/ Mo**
C	Regional Center Costs	Basic Rate +	$ 2,376.00 ($ 78.06/ day)	**$ 3,229.00/ Mo**

D	Regional Center Costs	Basic Rate +	$ 2,610.00 ($ 85.74/ day)	**$ 3,463.00/ Mo**
E	Regional Center Costs	Basic Rate +	$ 2,861.00 ($ 93.99/ day)	**$ 3,714.00/ Mo**
F	Regional Center Costs	Basic Rate +	$ 3,110.00 ($102.17/ day)	**$ 3,963.00/ Mo**
G	Regional Center Costs	Basic Rate +	$ 3,405.00 ($111.86/ day)	**$ 4,258.00/ Mo**
H	Regional Center Costs	Basic Rate +	$ 3,717.00 ($122.11/ day)	**$ 4,570.00/ Mo**
I	Regional Center Costs	Basic Rate +	$ 4,156.00 ($ 136.53/ day	**$ 5,009.00/ Mo**
ICF-DDH-DDN				**Approx. Starting at $ 5,300+/ Mo.**
Day Program Centers			per day per consumer	**$ 45.00 to $75.00**

An Easy Guide On How to Establish Your First Residential Care Facility

Group Home Rates and Classification Levels

Rate Classification Levels		Standard Rates
RCL Levels	Point Ranges	Per Consumer/Month
Level 1	60	$ 1,454.00
Level 2	61-89	$ 1,835.00
Level 3	90-119	$ 2,210.00
Level 4	120-149	$ 2,589.00
Level 5	150-179	$ 2,966.00
Level 6	180-209	$ 3,344.00
Level 7	210-239	$ 3,323.00
Level 8	240-269	$ 4,102.00
Level 9	270-299	$ 4,479.00
Level 10	300-329	$ 4,858.00
Level 11	330-359	$ 5,234.00
Level 12	360-389	$ 5,613.00
Level 13	390-419	$ 5,994.00
Level 14	420- UP	$ 6,371.00

(Rate may vary and subject to change without notice: January 2004)

Now that you have a general idea how much you are expecting to earn for your services, the next step is to create a business plan based on the figures presented to conduct the feasibility of the undertaking. But, before you do that, it is a good idea to first attend the initial orientation course sponsored by your local community care licensing office which is discussed on the next chapter.

Chapter 3: THE ORIENTATION

Step 1: Attend the 8 Hour Initial Orientation Sponsored by Your Local Community Care Licensing Office

The first important thing to do for start up individuals like you is to attend the initial orientation sponsored by your local community care licensing office. However, if you are one of those who purchased this book during the orientation, then move on to the next step.

Normally, the orientation takes about eight (8) hours divided into the morning session and afternoon session that normally starts SHARPLY at 9:00 A.M. and end before 5:00 P.M. held at the Local Community Care Licensing Office or the State/Federal Buildings where most government agency offices are located. There are some agencies who are considering the reduction on the orientation hours to four (4) hours only, so please ask your local licensing for schedules. To those who have not attended the orientation yet, please refer to this section for a list of local community care licensing offices CCL nearest you and call for orientation schedule which is posted on a monthly basis. The CCL list provided here include information such as the addresses, contact persons and the designated counties they cover. Due to continuing changes in area codes and zip codes, please check your local phone directory for current information on the addresses and contact numbers of these agencies.

During the orientation, most common topics to be discussed may vary from county to county and from agency to another. However, they all share one common format to the public which is to provide generalized information about the business. Here are some of the typical topics covered:

(a). Description of the types of facilities.
(b). The licensing requirements and processes.
(c). The expectations.
(d). The Regulation affecting the business etc...

The topics are divided into different sections and are discussed summarily just for the attendees to have a broad idea about the business. Later on when the attendees show interest and pursue the next level/stage, more information will be readily available through the licensing offices and based on individual readings and research on the business.

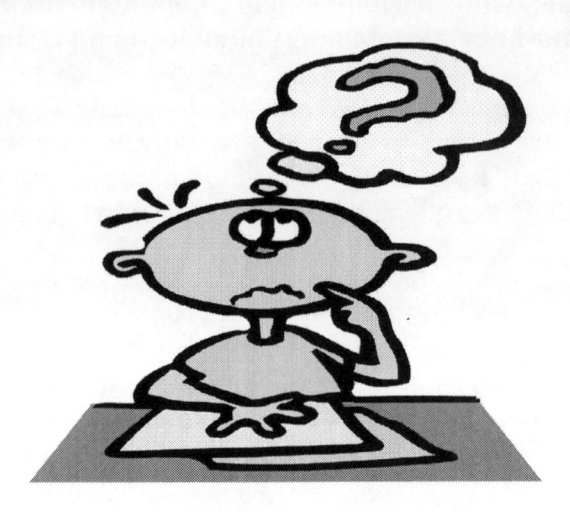

A. THE THREE COMPONENTS OF THE APPLICATION PROCESS

The Affidavit: After the orientation, each participant is given a white card identified as an Affidavit indicating the date when and where the orientation took place and signed by the seminar instructor. The date reflected on the card marks the start date of the effective window period of approximately six (6) months in order for the participant to fully complete the initial application process. Within said six (6) month period, the applicant must be able to complete the application process consisting of *three components namely:*

Component One: Initial Orientation attendance (8Hours),
Component Two: Partial Completion of the requirements, Submission of Application for a License And Program Design, Initial Visits etc…
Component Three: Final Facility Inspection and Final Correction of Program Design, Approval and Issuance of a License to Operate a Facility

B. WHAT ARE THE DIFFERENT FORMS NEEDED TO COMPLETE THE APPLICATION

After the Initial Orientation, the applicant is required to contact the local Community Care Licensing office to secure the blue packet also known as "The Application". When the applicant meets the basic requirements of the application, a License to Operate a facility may be granted on a probationary basis for at least six months to one year regardless whether the applicant makes a partial or full completion of the licensing requirements.

Here is a list of the most common requirements that the applicant is expected to complete in order to get to the third stage/component. The complete list of items are standard in the application process for most residential care facilities like for adults, facilities for the elderly, the chronically ill and day programs. There is a minor difference in requirements for group homes, foster family homes, small family homes, foster family agency and transition homes. More on this subject will be discussed later in this chapter.

a. Application Form ☐
b. Application Processing Fee ☐
   (Depending on facility, number of beds etc..)
c. Establishment of the Corporation/ ☐
   Non-profit / For Profit
d. Franchise Tax / IRS ☐
e. Employment Identification Number ☐
f. Administrator Certificate ☐
g. Business license ☐
h. Bank Account and statement ☐
i. Certification of available funds from the bank ☐
j. Health certificate, TB-HIV Test ☐
k. Live-Scan Fingerprint Clearances ☐
l. Facility / House ☐
m. Sketch ☐
n. Emergency Plan ☐
o. Disaster Plan ☐
p. Emergency Intervention Plan ☐
q. Business Forms ☐
r. Operations manual ☐

s. Business location ☐
t. Fire Marshall Certificate ☐
u. Host Letter ☐
v. Bonds ☐
w. General and Professional Liability insurance ☐
x. Transportation ☐
y. Program Design ☐
z. Staff ☐

These are just some of the standard requirements that one must be able to complete in time to expedite the application process. Check off any completed item as you go along and once these requirements are met accordingly and the application is submitted to the licensing office, the third stage is for the designated Licensing Program Analyst to conduct a site visit to verify the facility condition, available resources within the area and to complete the application process. The facility site must meet the standard of safety and should be ready for occupancy/operation at the time of visit. If the site requires further review, a corrective action plan will be issued by the visiting analyst and to schedule approximate date of completion of missing items. If the facility does not require further visit or site modification, a formal letter of acknowledgement will be provided to indicate facility license approval. Within fifteen (15) to thirty (30) days depending on the type of facility and client population to serve and if no pending licensing issue, a License to Operate a Facility will be issued to effect business operations. The expiration period indicated on the affidavit shall include the assumption that the applicant under went the whole application process which includes the completion of a program design, procurement of a facility and the applicants' ability to comply with the requirements set by the state regulation. Sometimes, the expiration may refer to the actual time frame when the applicant should be able to initiate and submit his application and not necessarily able to fully complete the process. If for any reason, the applicant is unable to meet the requirements on the last day of the expiration date as stated on the Affidavit, the applicant may possibly be permitted to request for an extension for the Affidavit if the licensing representative deems appropriate. But, it is not always the case when an applicant is granted an extension, otherwise, the applicant will be required to repeat the orientation sessions over again.

In completing the application packet, here are some important pointers to consider:

In order for a license to be issued, the licensing agency must review the information that is presented and that the applicant must meet the requirements for the license. As soon as the forms are complete, the application process is divided into two sections: **Section A and Section B**

SECTION A. GUIDELINES:

You must be able to submit the following items to the corresponding licensing agency:

- Group Home Application (Lic. 200) ☐
- Applicant Information (Lic. 215) ☐
- Designation of Administrative Responsibility (Lic. 308) ☐
- Administrative Organization (Lic. 309) ☐
- Affidavit regarding Client Cash Resources (Lic 400) ☐
- Estimated Monthly Operating Budget (Lic. 401) ☐
- Surety Bond (Lic. 402) ☐
- Financial Statement (Lic. 403) ☐
- Financial Information Release and Verification (Lic. 404) ☐
- Personnel Report (Lic. 500) ☐
- Personnel Record (Lic. 501) ☐
- Health Screening Report (Lic. 503) ☐
- Emergency Disaster Plan (Lic. 610) ☐
- Fingerprint Cards (BID 7A) ☐
- Child Abuse Index Check (Lic. 198A) ☐
- Facility Sketch (Lic. 999) ☐

All these information must be filed with the corresponding licensing agency that supervises the given area and will be reviewed by a designated licensing program analyst before a license may be issued. As soon as the licensing representative finds everything in order, applicant must file with the Department of Social Services within 60 days the remaining information that is requested for completion which includes the following:

- Articles of Incorporation ☐
- Verification of Facility Administrator ☐
- Verification of Social Worker qualification. ☐
- Job Description ☐
- Personnel Policies ☐
- In-Service Staff Training ☐
- Facility Program ☐
- Rules of Discipline ☐
- Admission Policies ☐
- Sample Menu ☐
- Control of Property ☐
- Bacteriological analysis ☐

The applicant must read the application carefully to make sure each question is understood thoroughly. The form must be filled out completely. If a corporation is applying for the license, it must indicate the applicant(s) corporate name. If a corporation is applying for the license, all persons signing the application must be authorized to do so as indicated in a Board Resolution. All applicants must sign the application, including each general partner. The application shall have original signatures only and no photo-copies allowed. The signatures need to match the applicant's name unless the application is a corporation. If the application indicates that the applicant previously held a license for a facility, check to make sure that this is also reflected on the Applicant Information (LIC 215). There will be a verification that no disciplinary action was or is pending on any previously or currently licensed facility.

LIC. 215 APPLICANT INFORMATION.

Make sure that the form is completed by each applicant. If the applicant previously held a license, held a beneficial ownership of 10 percent or more or was an administrator, general partner, corporate officer or director of a licensed facility, research to determine if any disciplinary actions were or are being taken. LIC. FORM No. 215 can be used, as necessary, to verify qualifications when an applicant also intends to be the Administrator/Director.

LIC. 308 DESIGNATION OF ADMINISTRATIVE RESPONSIBILITY

This form must contain the original signature(s) of the Applicant(s)/Licensee(s) and must not be photocopied. If an individual other than the licensee is designated as the administrator/director or other agent of the facility to act on behalf of the absent licensee or if the applicant is a corporation, there must be a Board Resolution authorizing the delegation of responsibility.

LIC. 309 ADMINISTRATIVE ORGANIZATION

This form must be filled out if the applicant is a Corporation, Public Agency, Partnership or other Association. Make sure this information matches the information which appears on the Application (LIC. 200).

LIC. 400 AFFIDAVIT REGARDING CLIENT CASH RESOURCES

It must be signed and completed and the appropriate box is checked. In most cases when the facility holds client funds, a bond must be applied for by the applicant.

Situations when a bond is needed:

1. The licensee/facility employee cashes a client's check at the bank and returns the money to the client.
2. The licensee/facility employee handles the client's money.
3. The licensee/facility employee keeps client money in a safe place, including a bank/financial institution, and controls its distribution ("hands out the money").

(Not applicable in Day Care Centers or Foster Family Agencies)

LIC. 402 SURETY BOND

The bonding agency may use the language found on the LIC. 402, if the form itself is not used. The State of California must be identified as the Principal (recipient) and there must be an effective date and an expiration date.

THE FOLLOWING FINANCIAL FORMS ARE NECESSARY IN ORDER TO CAPTURE THE OVERALL FINANCIAL STATUS OF THE APPLICANT AND TO DETERMINE IF THE APPLICANT HAS SUFFICIENT FINANCIAL RESOURCES TO OPERATE THE FACILITY (I.E., MEET EXPENSES). THESE FORMS WILL BE REVIEWED IN CONJUNCTION WITH ONE ANOTHER, AS WELL AS WITH A CREDIT REPORT, IF ONE HAS BEEN OBTAINED.

LIC. 401 ESTIMATED MONTHLY OPERATING BUDGET

The number of clients corresponds with the requested capacity. Other income must be clear and documented. All operating costs must be indicated and reasonable (i.e., salaries are shown at least minimum wage). Approximately 25 percent of the salaries shall normally be added for fringe benefits. If fringe benefits are not applicable, the application should so state and explained why. The rent amount corresponds with the lease/rental agreement/mortgage payment. If the applicant is the licensee of any other facility, an LIC. 401 must also be submitted for each licensed facility. This information must reflect the actual operating budget, not an estimate (The word "Estimated" found on the top of the LIC. 401 should be lined out and replaced with "Actual" for each currently licensed facility).

LIC. 403 FINANCIAL STATEMENT

The information to be provided must reflect assets and liabilities concerning all activities of the owner(s), not just those related to the operation of the facility (i.e., credit card balances, income and expenses related to other businesses). The figures provided must be "Realistic." Life insurance amount must be the cash value or surrender value not "face value" (normally the amount to be paid upon death). If the applicant is the sole owner, real estate listed should indicate appraised value of property. If the applicant is a partnership or corporation, the cost of the real estate should be indicated not the appraised value. On-site furnishings and equipment listed should indicate the appraised value. Funds/assets must be readily available to the facility (i.e., not dependent upon the sale or transfer of stock or personal property).

NOTE: The credit report can be used to verify that liabilities have been fully disclosed.

LIC. 404 FINANCIAL INFORMATION RELEASE AND VERIFICATION

(One form or set of forms is required for each amount.) The applicant must complete Section 1 and return the form to the licensing agency. The licensing agency shall send this form to the financial institution. The verification must be sent by the financial institution directly to the licensing agency. The licensee cannot hand carry it. This information is used to verify approximately three months of operating budget (cross referenced to the estimated monthly operating budget). The licensing agency will take into account situations such as the following:

1. The applicant is purchasing an already licensed and operational facility.
2. Portions of the start-up funds have been spent on start-up costs (i.e., repairs to meet fire safety).
3. Clients/children are enrolled and/or a waiting list has been established.

A verifiable "line of credit" from a reputable financial institution is acceptable for start-up funds, if readily accessible.

LIC. 420 BUDGET INFORMATION

(To be completed by Small Family Home Applicants also) Must contain original signature(s), cannot be photocopied.

LIC. 500 PERSONNEL REPORT

(Separate form is required for each day care component.) All positions are to be shown on this form with days and hours on duty. Make sure there is the required staff coverage for all hours of operation. Director/Administrator and any teachers/staff hired at the time of application should be on the form. Other positions with staff not yet hired must be listed as "to be hired" and designated by position title. If the form does not show that the director/administrator is there full time, a qualified substitute must be designated (i.e., in a day care center if the director is not opening and closing the facility, a qualified substitute must do so). Make sure anyone designated as exempt from fingerprinting requirements is appropriate pursuant to Health and Safety Code Sections 1522, 1569.17 and 1596.871 and that Side B is signed by the applicant/licensee or designated representative (signature(s) cannot be photocopied). Make sure all persons required to be fingerprinted have submitted fingerprint cards (BID 7B).

LIC. 501 PERSONNEL RECORD

This form is to be signed and submitted to the licensing agency only for Director/Administrator and Program Manager, if required. All others are to be kept on file for review at the facility. Verification of education and experience will be done against official school transcripts and/or references.

LIC. 503 HEALTH SCREENING REPORT

(This form is not required, under certain circumstances, of persons who are adherents of a well-recognized church relying solely upon prayer or spiritual means of healing. Facilities must, however, present satisfactory evidence to the licensing agency that individuals are free from any communicable disease. Such evidence shall be a written statement from a practitioner recognized by this religion for the purposes of healing.) One form or set of forms each is required for the applicant and the director. Health screening, at time of application, must be less than six months old for applicants for Residential Care Facilities for the Elderly and one year old for all other categories. (If the applicant has other licensed facilities, or the director has worked at another facility with the same licensee, and there is an exam on file, a new health exam is not required unless there are obvious health problems.) If the applicant is a corporation, there must be a health screening with a TB clearance for the Board President, Chief Executive Officer or person designated by the Board Resolution.

LIC. 503 TB Test

The form must be signed and dated by a qualified medical professional (signature(s) cannot be photocopied). The TB test portion of the form must be filled out, including result, or a separate test verification is needed.

LIC. 610 or LIC, 610A EMERGENCY DISASTER PLAN

(A separate form is required for each component of a day care program.) The plan must show a relocation site away from the facility that is able to accommodate the number of clients/children in the facility. If the use of the relocation site requires an agreement from some other agency or person, make sure this is verified in writing.

BID 7A FINGERPRINT CARD

Fingerprinting is required for all applicant(s), administrator/director, and residents (other than clients) except those designated exempt (see Health and Safety Code Sections 1522, 1596.871 and 1569.17). Fingerprinting clearance is required on all new staff before initial contacts with the consumers unless previously cleared with another facility and currently on active status. Fingerprint clearance must be received on the applicant(s), administrator/director and all adults (except clients) living in the facility prior to licensure. Fingerprint processing fees must be included, when required. Each box checked on the BID 7A must be completed. With most agencies using LIVE-Scan fingerprinting, copies of fingerprinting results must be on file prior to initial contact with the clients at the facility.

LIC. 198A CHILD ABUSE INDEX CHECK

(Applies to all facilities serving children.) LIC 198As are required for the applicant(s), administrator/director, and residents (other than clients) who are associated with a facility serving children and are required to be fingerprinted. LIC 198 Should be submitted to DOJ as new staff are hired. Child Abuse Index Checks must be received on the applicant(s), administrator/director and all adults (except clients) living in the facility prior to licensure. Child Abuse Index Checks are mailed directly to DOJ along with a $15.00 processing fee. Child Abuse Index Checks and Fingerprint Cards should be submitted together. With the introduction of on-site live scan fingerprinting process, an individual person may be fingerprinted at any local designated fingerprinting agency for about $ 45.00 which shall cover cost for fingerprinting, child abuse index and DOJ notification. The process shall take within less thirty minutes.

LIC. 999 FACILITY SKETCH

Sketch must give dimensions of all rooms and designate their use. Rooms to be used by non-ambulatory clients/residents should be identified. A facility sketch is required for all indoor and outdoor space including driveways, fences, storage areas, gardens, recreation areas and other space used by clients/residents. For Day Care Centers, submit separate sketches for indoor and outdoor space for each component and one sketch showing entire facility and relationship between indoor and outdoor spaces of all components, as well as any other use of the building. Sketch of outdoor space/ playground must show dimensions and location of major equipment and swimming pools.

SECTION B GUIDELINES

The following guidelines are used when reviewing application documents for Section B. Within the section below you will find some items that are less detailed than others. This is because the California Code of Regulations (CCR) section identified below the criteria is either self-explanatory when read or is quite specific and/ or lengthy. Therefore, when developing and reviewing each Section

B document it is necessary to refer to the CCR (regulation) section listed in order to fully understand the regulatory requirement. It should also be kept in mind that the application document review is only one portion of the application decision-making process. Findings from the pre-licensing visit may prohibit approval of the application because of physical plant or other deficiencies which are not specific elements of the application document package.

1. Articles of Incorporation

The Articles of Incorporation are used to prove that the applicant is in fact a legitimate corporation and approved to do business as such in the State of California. The articles should include a state seal from the state in which they are incorporated. This indicates that it is a valid corporation. Out-of-state/foreign corporations are automatically authorized to operate in California. (In these cases, all of the information required below is still needed.) Pursuant to regulations, the following information must be provided as part of, or in support of, the Articles of Incorporation:

2. Constitution and By laws

This is reviewed only to ensure that no licensing regulations are violated. Board Resolution to determine who are the agents acting on behalf of the corporation. Authorization to apply for a license and the person authorized and delegated by Board Resolution to sign and act on behalf of the corporation should be included in the board resolution. This may be the Chief Executive Officer, Board President, Board member, or an individual from the Corporate Executive Office. Board Officers' names, titles, business and home addresses and phone numbers.

3. Verification of Administrator / Director Qualifications

Administrator/director qualifications and duties are found in licensing regulations. When applicable, these requirements must be verified by the following means by the applicant/licensee and provided to the licensing agency as part of Section B.

Education: Transcripts from an accredited school (Courses can be compared to the Early Childhood Education (ECE) matrix for verification of acceptance) or a copy of the Children's Center Supervisory Permit.

Out-of-country school: In order to determine that the appropriate classes and numbers of units have been completed, the applicant/licensee should obtain a copy of the class description(s) or college catalog describing the class or obtain verification from a local college regarding class equivalency.

Experience: If required, written references are to be obtained by the applicant/licensee and submitted to the licensing agency. References are to include the following information required by regulation: Each year of experience shall be verified as having been performed satisfactorily, at least 3 hours per day for a minimum of 100 days in a calendar year, as a teacher under the supervision of a person who would qualify as a director under these regulations.

Job Descriptions: As part of the operation of the facility, the applicant must establish staff positions that will be responsible for specific tasks or duties. The applicant must provide the licensing agency with a job description for each of these classifications. The description needs to be clear, concise and relevant to the position for which the person is being hired. Additionally, job descriptions will be compared to the Personnel Report (LIC. 500) and there must be a job description for each classification listed on the LIC 500.

Duties and Responsibilities: Minimum Qualifications that correspond to licensing requirements. This is to include any special licenses or certificates, if they are required by the profession.) Special skills needed to perform the job. Lines of supervision: (This is to include supervision given to and from whom, as well as, supervision received and from whom).

4. Personnel Policies

Personnel policies are to describe those regulatory requirements commonly associated with personnel practices/policies such as staff coverage, staff qualification, work schedules and conditions of employment. The following areas are to be included in this section.

1. Work hours/shifts for documentation of positions to provide coverage with competent staff.

2. Employee rights. (A statement that employees are to be informed of their rights will suffice).

3. Abuse reporting procedures. Documentation must indicate that employees will be informed of their responsibilities to report to the licensing agency as well as to the child/adult protective agency.

4. Hiring practices; including screening of employees for necessary education and experience and informing employees that conditions of their employment include fingerprint clearance, statement of prior criminal convictions, TB clearance, physical examination/health questionnaire, child abuse index check. (This is to ensure that employees are competent and aware that they have to meet these conditions for initial and continued employment.)

5. Other federal and state agencies have requirements that businesses must adhere to in relation to personnel practices, such as, minimum wages, Workmen's Compensation and Fair Employment Practices. These agencies monitor the business's compliance with their regulations. Community Care Licensing does not enforce other agencies' regulations. It is important, however, that applicants contact these agencies in order to determine that established practices are not in conflict with laws or regulations

5. In-Service Training for Staff

As part of the plan of operation of the facility, the applicant must establish a plan for in-service training for staff and submit the plan to the licensing agency at the time of application. The plan must address the following:

(a). Staff will receive training (new staff versus on-going staff) and indicate how it is determined which staff will receive training, and who will do the training.

(b). Topics to be covered in the training. (This is to be reviewed in order to ensure that the topics covered are pertinent to the facility/client type and the duties performed.)

6. Facility Program Description

The Program Description should be a general overview of the program philosophies, goals, basic and optional services and activities to be provided by the applicant. This can be explained as to what the public would want to know about the facility and could be used as an advertisement for the facility. A pamphlet or brochure advertising the facility is also acceptable providing all of the following elements:

(a). Child Care Program Description: Brief statement of the purpose, goals and program methods. (Information on specific philosophies, if any.)

(b). Schedule of daily activities to include:

1. Day and hours of operation.
2. Times that meals and snacks are served.
3. Nap time (if required).
4. Times of specific activities.

The Program Description should also contain information outlined in the "Admission Policies" section of the regulations:

1. Designation of children/consumers whose needs can be met by the center's program.
2. Ages of children/consumers accepted.
3. Supplementary services, if any.
4. Field trip provisions, if any.
5. Transportation arrangements, if any.
6. Food services provisions (description must clearly indicate who will provide optional food services for each meal and whether food will be prepared in the facility or brought in from an outside source).
7. Indicate whether medications will be administered to children. A separate plan for medications must be

developed if the licensee elects to handle medications (over-the-counter or prescription).
8. Information regarding consultant and community resources to be utilized as part of the program, particularly detailed for programs serving children with special needs.) This must be services to be provided if a child has a medical or dental emergency. Sign-in and sign-out procedures - the licensee must have a written procedure for transfer of responsibility between the center and the parent or guardian.

7. Discipline Policies:

The applicant shall describe the type(s) of discipline that will be used and under what conditions each type will be used. The discipline policies shall also address the following, when appropriate:

1. Types of discipline not permitted.
   NO CORPORAL PUNISHMENT OR VIOLATION OF PERSONAL RIGHTS

2. Provisions for contact with parents/placement representatives (conferences) Grounds for dismissal / eviction / relocation / removal from placement.

NOTE: Prone containment and like techniques shall not be included as part of the facility's discipline policy nor written into individual client's needs and services plan. Such techniques are not to be a planned step in modifying behavior. They are considered to be only last resort emergency physical control techniques designed to prevent injury to bystanders, the assaultive client, other clients, and staff. The Department will evaluate the discipline policies to ensure that these policies do not violate personal rights and that there is a clear statement that there will be no corporal or unusual punishment used. If there is reason to believe that the applicant does not understand what constitutes corporal punishment or a violation of personal rights, or the statements have not been made clear, then further information may be requested.

8. Admission Policies:

The admission policies must provide information relevant to the category and types of consumers accepted for care, ages of the clients, rates and refund policies, acceptance and retention limitations, pre-admission appraisals, needs and services plans, medical assessments and an Admission Agreement which contains the typical information a consumer or his or her authorized representative would need to know prior to entering a facility. A description of the following items must be included in this section:

1. Persons accepted for care, including age range and compatibility determination process, when necessary.

2. Intake procedures for placement in Group Homes.

3. Criteria for determining appropriateness of placement given individual client's needs (i.e.) interviews, procedures for obtaining and developing the necessary paperwork).

4. Needs and Services Plan.

5. Client's Rights/Personal Rights. (At a minimum there should be a statement that clients/residents will be informed of their rights and that client's/resident's rights will not be violated).

6. Medical Assessment.

7. Pre-Admission Appraisal Plan.

8. Emergency Information.

9. Sign-in and Sign-out Procedures.

10. Immunization Requirements.

11. Physical Examination Requirements (including TB testing).

12. Admission Agreement. The admission agreement is to include the following information. (The Department's Admission Agreement Guide (LIC 604 or LIC 604A) is an acceptable form which covers the areas necessary for residential facilities.):

- Description of basic services offered. (All basic services must be either offered or, if a client is currently obtaining specific services through other means, planned for in the event the service is needed at a future date.)

- Description of optional services offered. (Reviewed to ensure that required "Basic Services" are not included in this description).

- Payment provisions, such as rates for basic & optional services, payor, due date, and frequency of payments. (Reviewed to ensure provisions are clear and rate charged to SSI/SSP recipients does not exceed the established maximum).

- Modification conditions. (Reviewed to ensure at least 30 day advanced notice for rate change).

- Refund Policy. (Reviewed to ensure that the policy is clear and is not in violation of licensing regulations).

- Rights of the licensing agency.

- Reasons for termination. (Reviewed to ensure that this section is not in violation of licensing regulations).

- Visiting policy.

- House rules.

9. Sample Menu:

It is important for the licensing agency to verify that the applicant is familiar with the provision of balanced meals, acceptable portion sizes and general principles of good nutrition. A sample menu is needed in order to meet this requirement. The sample menu will include:

- 1 week's worth of planned meals (to include snacks) from the four basic food groups.

- Portion sizes. Evaluate portion sizes using the handbook section found in the regulations.

- Time meals served. (Reviewed for time elapsed between last meal of the day and first meal of the next day.)

10. Control of Property:

It is necessary for the licensing agency to determine that the applicant/licensee has control over the property that is being or is to be used as a facility. Once licensed, the licensee must be able to ensure that the facility and grounds are maintained and are in compliance with regulations (i.e., repairs made to the physical plan, fences around swimming pools, etc.).

- Name and address of the owner must be provided.

- A copy of the lease agreement or rental agreement must be provided. (There are no requirements related to length of the lease or rental agreement.) If the agreement precludes the use of the property as a facility, prevents the applicant/licensee from achieving compliance with regulations, or the operation of a facility is contrary to the terms of the agreement, the license must be denied/withdrawn as the licensee would not have adequate control over the property (i.e., the agreement states that Susie and Mary are to be the persons residing in the house and anyone else needs to be approved, the agreement states the property cannot be used for business purposes and the applicant wishes to operate a facility for more than 6 persons).

- Proof of Ownership must be provided if the applicant is the owner of the property. This is verified by a Deed or Property Tax bill.

11. Bacterial Analysis of Water:

This is required for all categories at initial licensure if water for consumption is from a private source, regardless of the number of clients served. Submit evidence of on-site inspection of the source of the water and a bacteriological analysis by a local or state health department or other qualified laboratory which establishes the safety of the water. If the analysis provided gives only a chemical/ bacteriological analysis and not a specific statement as to whether or not the water is safe to drink, request that the applicant get such a statement from the laboratory. The analysis must be signed by a qualified agency representative.

On the following pages is the list of community care licensing offices that you will need to call for the schedule of orientation, information on licensing requirements and procedures.

DEPARTMENT OF SOCIAL SERVICES
744 P Street, Sacramento, CA. 95814

Technical Support (916) 229-4500 RCFE Certification Unit (916) 324-4031

COMMUNITY CARE LICENSING DIVISION FIELD OFFICES

NORTHERN REGIONAL OFFICE
8745 Folsom Blvd. Suite 130. M.S. 19-48
Sacramento, CA 95826
(916) 229-4500   FAX (916) 229-4508

CHICO DISTRICT -RESIDENTIAL AND CHILD CARE
520 Cabaret Road, Suite 6, M.S,29-05
Manager: Earl Nance
Chico, CA 95926
(530) 895-5033FAX (530) 895-5934
Counties: Butte, Colusa. Del None, Glenn. Humbolt, Lassen, Modoc, Plumas, Shasta, Sierra, Siskiyou, Sutter, Tehama, Trinity and Yuba

SACRAMENTO DISTRICT - RESIDENTIAL
2400 Glendale Lane, Suite C, M.S. 19-35
 Manager: Gary Levenson-Palmer,   Sacramento, CA 95825
(916) 574-2346FAX (916) 574-2382
Counties: Amador, Calaveras, El Dorado, Nevada. Placer,
Sacramento, San Joaquin. Stanislaus, Tuolumne and Yolo

SACRAMENTO DISTRICT - CHIILD CARE
8745 Folsom Blvd., Suite 200, M.S. 19-29
Manager: Charles Boatman, Sacramento, CA 95826
(916) 229-4530FAX (916) 387-1933
Counties : Alpine, Amador, Calaveras, El Dorado, Nevada, Placer,
Sacramento, San Joaquin, Stanislaus, Tolumne and Yolo

REDWOOD EMPIRE DISTRICT - RESIDENTIAL & CHILD CARE
101 Golf Course Drive. Suite A-230, M.S. 29-11
Manager: Wayne Wilson, Rohnert Park, CA 94928 (707) 585-5026
FAX (707) 588-5080 Counties: Lake, Marin, Mendocino, Napa,
Solano, and Sonoma

FRESNO DISTRICT -RESIDENTIAL AND CHILD CARE
770 E. Shaw Avenue, Suite 330. M.S. 29-0
Manager: Dave Guinan Fresno, CA 93710
(209) 445 3691   FAX (209) 445-5097
Counties: Alpine, Fresno. Inyo, Kern, Kings, Madera Mariposa.
Merced, Mono and Tulare

COASTAL REGIONAL OFFICE
801 Traeger Ave., Suite 105, M.S. 29-18
Manager: Martha Mills
San Bruno, CA 94066   (650) 266-8860
FAX (650) 266-8877

CENTRAL COAST AREA - RESIDENTIAL AND CHILD CARE
360 S. Hope Avenue, Suite C-105, M.S. 29-09
Manager: Joseph Brocato
Santa Barbara, CA 93105   (805) 682-7647
FAX (805) 682-8361
Counties: San Luis Obispo, Santa Barbara and Ventura

BAY AREA DISTRICT- CHILD CARE
200 Webster Street, Suite 100. M.S. 29-04
Manager: .Melissa Miller
Oakland, CA 94607 (510) 286-7062
FAX   (510) 286-7113
Counties: Alameda and Contra Costa

PENINSULA DISTRICT -CHILD CARE
801 Traeger Avenue. Suite I00, M.S. 29-24
Manager: Fred Gill
San Bruno, CA 94066   (650) 266-8843
FAX   (650) 266-8847
Counties: San Francisco and San Mateo

An Easy Guide On How to Establish Your First Residential Care Facility

SAN FRANCISCO BAY - RESIDENTIAL
851 Traeger Avenue, Suite 360. M.S. 29-16
Manager: Stan Roman
San Bruno. CA 94066   (650) 266-8800
FAX (650) 266-8841
Counties: Alameda, Contra Costa, San Francisco and
San .Mateo

SAN JOSE DISTRICT - CHILD CARE
111 North Market Street. Suite 300. M.S. 29-08
Manager: Gary Baysmore
San Jose. CA 95113   (408) 277-1286
FAX   (408) 277-2071
Counties: Monterey. San Benito, Santa Clara and Santa Cruz

SAN JOSE DISTRICT-RESIDENTIAL
111 North Market Street. Suite 350. M.S. 29-07
Manager : Barbara Murdy
San Jose. CA. 95113   (408) 277-1289
FAX (408) 277-2045
Counties: Monterey. San Benito. Santa Clara and Santa Cruz

SOUTHERN REGIONAL OFFICE
5962 La Place Court. Suite 185 M.S. 29-19
Carlsbad. CA. 92008   (760) 929-2121
FAX (760) 929-2133

MISSION VALLEY DISTRICT - CHILD CARE
8765 Aero Drive, Suite 300, M.S. 29-20
Manager: Terry Sutton
San Diego, CA. 92123   (619) 467-4388
FAX (619) 492-1755
County: San Diego, Imperial

SAN DIEGO DISTRICT- RESIDENTIAL
8745 Aero Drive, Suite 200,M.S. 29-06
Manager: Mary Delmast
San Diego. CA. 92123   (619) 467-2367
FAX (619) 467-2373
Counties: Imperial and San Diego

SAN GORGONIO OFFICE - CHILD CARE
3737 Main Street. Suite 700. M.S. 29-12
Manager: Mary Kaarwaa
Riverside. CA 92501   (909) 782-4200
FAX (909) 782-4985
Counties: Riverside and San Bernardino

INLAND EMPIRE OFFICE - RESIDENTIAL
3737 Main Street. Suite 600. M.S. 29-26
Manager: Robert Gonzales
Riverside, CA. 92501   (909) 782-4207
FAX (909) 782-4967
Counties: Riverside and San Bernardino

ORANGE COUNTY- CHILD CARE
750 The City Drive. Suite 250, M.S. 29-I0
Manager: Arthur Carter
Orange, CA 92668   (714) 703-2800
FAX (714) 703-2831
County: Orange

ORANGE COUNTY - RESIDENTIAL
770 The City Drive. Suite 7100. M.S. 29-28
Manager: Bob Gomez
Orange, CA. 92668   (714) 703-2840
FAX (714) 703-2868
County: Orange

LOS ANGELES REGIONAL OFFICE
100 Corporate Point, Suite 350. M.S. 29-17
Culver City. CA 90230   (310) 665-1940
FAX   (310) 665-1979

L. A. RESIDENTIAL EAST
1000 Corporate Center Drive. Suite 200-A. M.S. 3 I0
Manager: Robert Pate, Monterey Park. CA 91754
(213) 981-3100   FAX (213) 981-3309

L.A. RESIDENTIAL - NORTHERN VALLEYS
21731 Ventura Blvd., Suite 250. M.S. 29-14
Manager: Joana Hirai
Woodland Hills. CA. 91364   (818) 596-4334
FAX (818) 596-4376

L. A. RESIDENTIAL WEST
6167 Bristol Parkway. 1210, M.S. 31-09
Manager: Lydia Thomas Culver City,   CA 90230
(310) 568-1807   FAX (310) 417.3680

L.A. NORTHWEST - CHILD CARE
6167 Bristol Parkway. 1400. M.S. 29-13
Manager: Sergio Ramirez
Culver City. CA 90230   (310) 337-4333
FAX (310) 337-4360

L.A. CHILD CARE EAST
1000 Corporate Center Drive. Suite 20O-B. M.S. 29-15
Manager: Lois Petzold, Monterey Park, CA. 91754
(213) 981-3350   FAX (213) 981-3355

ORANGE COUNTY - RESIDENTIAL
770 The City Drive. Suite 7100. M.S. 29-28
Manager: Bob Gomez
Orange, CA. 92668   (714) 703-2840
FAX (714) 703-2868
County: Orange

An Easy Guide On How to Establish Your First Residential Care Facility

LOS ANGELES REGIONAL OFFICE
100 Corporate Point, Suite 350. M.S. 29-17
Culver City. CA 90230   (310) 665-1940
FAX   (310) 665-1979

L. A. RESIDENTIAL EAST
1000 Corporate Center Drive. Suite 200-A. M.S. 3 I0
Manager: Robert Pate, Monterey Park. CA 91754
(213) 981-3100   FAX (213) 981-3309

L.A. RESIDENTIAL - NORTHERN VALLEYS
21731 Ventura Blvd., Suite 250. M.S. 29-14
Manager: Joana Hirai
Woodland Hills. CA. 91364   (818) 596-4334
FAX (818) 596-4376

L. A. RESIDENTIAL WEST
6167 Bristol Parkway. 1210, M.S. 31-09
Manager: Lydia Thomas Culver City,   CA 90230
(310) 568-1807   FAX (310) 417.3680

L.A. NORTHWEST - CHILD CARE
6167 Bristol Parkway. 1400. M.S. 29-13
Manager: Sergio Ramirez
Culver City. CA 90230   (310) 337-4333

FAX (310) 337-4360

L.A. CHILD CARE EAST
1000 Corporate Center Drive. Suite 20O-B. M.S. 29-15
Manager: Lois Petzold, Monterey Park, CA. 91754
(213) 981-3350   FAX (213) 981-3355

ORIENTATION AFFIDAVIT
(Sample)

State of California-Health and Welfare Agency   Dept. of Social Services

ORIENTATION/APPLICATION PROCESS
CERTIFICATE OF COMPLETION

_____
Name of Applicant

COMPONENT I CATEGORY SPECIFIC ORIENTATION SESSION

Date Attended	District office	Facility Category	Evaluator's Signature

COMPONENT II – FACE TO FACE INTERVIEW

Date Attended	Person Attending	Job Title	Evaluator's Signature

Date Attended	Person Attending	Job Title	Evaluator's Signature

COMPONENT III CATEGORY SPECIFIC ORIENTATION/TRAINING

Date Attended	District office	Facility Category	Evaluator's Signature

Effective Date of License _____   Authorized Signature _____

Lic 281 C (7/92)

Chapter 4: THE FACILITY ADMINISTRATOR CERTIFICATION COURSE

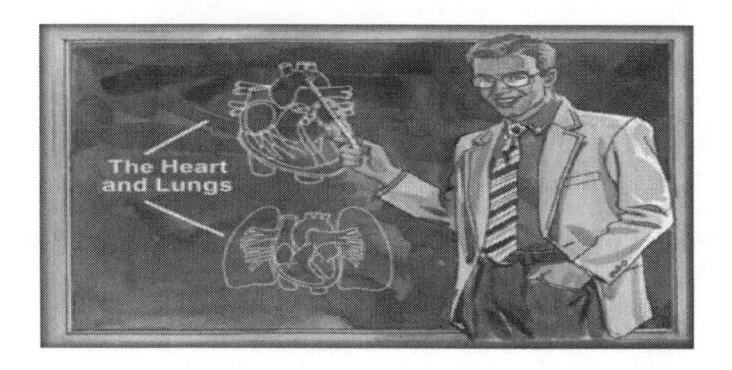

Step 2. BECOME A CERTIFIED FACILITY ADMINISTRATOR

Take the Facility Administrator Initial Certification Course

The second plan of action is to become a certified facility administrator. No one is better qualified to run the business other than the owner himself. As the owner, you need to know how your business runs and not rely solely on someone else. Every residential care facility (including day programs) must have a certified administrator. You can become a certified administrator upon completion of the required training hours that typically last for at least 40 Hours for Group Home Administrators and Administrators for Residential Care Facility for the Elderly and other facilities. Meanwhile, 35 Hours of Certification Training is required for Adult Residential Care Facility Administrators. To be able to take the class, the applicant must enroll with a vendorized training instructor/provider normally found in the list of accredited training providers approved by the local Community Care Licensing office. These training providers are mostly private instructors who by their education and experience in the field and in the business qualify as certified instructors of the standardized certification courses set forth by Community Care Licensing.

Are you allowed to take classes from Universities or Vocational schools/Colleges offering these certification courses?

If the school is vendorized and appears on the list of accredited providers by the licensing agency, YES. If they do not appear on the list, your certification course may not be considered valid which means that despite of the fact that you attended the required hours and received a certificate of completion, it does not mean you may be allowed to take the state exam. Only those recognized by the state to provide certification courses are allowed to teach and to issue certificates of course completion. By the way, the list is available through the local Community Care Licensing office who keeps track of who is currently vendorized and who is not.

As a future business owner of a residential care facility, is it a requirement that you as licensee must become a certified administrator in order to establish your residential care facility?

No. Being a licensee/owner is different from the role of being an administrator. You have the option to be or not to be. If for reasons, you, as the applicant /owner of the facility choose not to be the administrator, you have the option to hire a certified administrator to represent your company. Regardless of the type of the facility whether it be a residential care facility or a day program, there must be a Certified Administrator who will supervise and manage the facility's over-all operation. If one is to manage or become an administrator for two different types of homes/ facilities for example a residential care facility for children and another facility for seniors, the administrator is required to be certified for two separate certification courses, Group Home Administrator and Administrator for Residential Care Facility for the Elderly. As an administrator, you are allowed to manage a maximum of two group homes, while in residential care facilities for adults and the elderly, you may be allowed to manage more than two as long as the number of hours allocated in managing the facilities are within the allowable limits to properly execute your duties and responsibilities as administrator. (Check with your local licensing representative on this subject).

The general rule is that, to become an administrator, one must be at least 21 years of age (but for some states, must be at least 18), has the right to work in the US and must be of good moral and ethical character. All administrators must attend the required certification course and possess a certificate of attendance upon completion of the required certification hours. The certificate of completion issued by the accredited school where the participant attended will entitle the individual graduate of the course to qualify to take the state certification examination within 60-days from the date of issuance of the certificate of attendance.

Schedule yourself to attend the required hours for Initial Administrator Certification Course.

It is very helpful to attend the Initial Administrator Certification Course at first, before you do any major action related to your business because most of the topics in the course discussion are directly related to the business itself. You will realize later on that you will find a lot of useful information in the class that you can apply in your business plan, program design and operating procedures and policies. It is also a good source for fresh information on the type of facility you are contemplating on establishing and to know the latest information on the trends, as well as present and future plans of the state concerning the business.

Take the State Certification Exam and Pass it.

All residential care facilities must have a certified administrator. All facility administrators are required to be state certified before assuming the official role of an administrator. In order to be certified, an individual must take the state sponsored certification exam and must pass it within 60 days after graduating from state vendorized schools/instructors. It is very important to take the state exam with a passing score of 70% or better in order to receive a congratulatory letter. If the test taker fails the exam and has exceeded beyond the regulatory 60-day period, he/she is required to repeat the class over again and must re-take the exam until he/she pass it.

When you take the test, and are unsure of the results of your effort, it is important that you create a plan on how to sequentially take the test more than once from at least two different testing sites in case you are considering possible re-takes. There is no limit as to how many times you will be allowed to take the test as long as you are able pass the test within 60 days from the date you complete the administrator certification class. So, plan a strategy on how you will take the test accordingly. The testing centers require no prior appointment in order to take the test, but you need to call for testing dates to prepare your schedule ahead of time. Be at the testing site at least one hour before the actual test to avoid the unexpected, reduce anxiety and your anxiousness to get it over with the test.

Upon receipt of a congratulatory letter indicating that you pass the test, you must send the following information as soon as possible:

1. A copy of a letter from the State indicating that you passed the test.

2. A copy of the certificate of completion of the administrator course.

3. Fingerprint clearance from FBI-DOJ through Live-Scan or a request for transfer of fingerprint clearance from previous employment.

4. A copy of your CPR-First Aid certification

5. HIV-Hepatitis certification (Optional)

6. Application Processing Fee

7. And other documentations that may be requested by Community Care Licensing office.

Send the documents by mail and expect a response within 30 to 60 days. By the way, the processing fee is non-refundable.

The Background Check Process

Everyone involved in the health care business either by profession or job related purpose is required to have a background check either by fingerprint or by other means.

The California Health and Safety Code requires a background check of all applicants, licensees, adult residents, volunteers under certain conditions and employees of community care facilities *who have contact with clients.* If the California Department of Social Services finds that an individual is convicted of a crime other than a minor traffic violation, he/she must not work or be present in any community care facility unless he/she is granted a criminal record exemption from the Community Care Licensing Division, Caregiver Background Check Bureau (CBCB). What is an exemption? Exemption is a Department authorized written document that "exempts" the individual from the requirement of having a criminal record clearance. CBCB also examines arrest records to determine if there is a possible danger to clients (Health & Safety Code Sections 1522, 1568.08, 1569.17, and 1596.871).

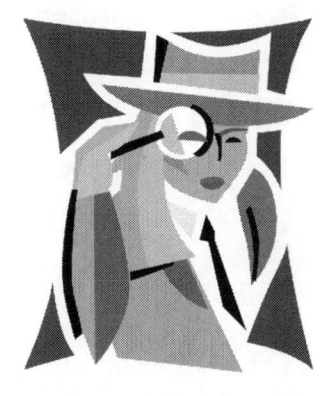

How is the Background Check Conducted?

When an individual submits fingerprints, the California Department of Justice (DOJ) conducts a background check. If the individual has no criminal history, DOJ will forward a clearance notice to the applicant or licensee and to CBCB. If the individual has a criminal history, DOJ will send a criminal record transcript to CBCB. The transcript will show arrests and convictions. CBCB staff will review the transcript and if the convictions are for crimes that may be exempted, CBCB will send an exemption notification letter to the applicant or licensee. The letter explains how to request an exemption and lists the documents/information that must be submitted together with the request. The individual may not be present at the facility until an exemption is granted by CBCB.

Child Abuse Central Index (CACI)

The Child Abuse Central Index name check is an additional background check required for individuals associated to any facility that cares for children. This requirement took effect in January 1, 1986. If the CACI check is required, an exemption can not be granted until this portion of the background check is also cleared. Effective January 1, 1999, the Department of Justice now provides

CBCB with notification of any subsequent incidents of child abuse after the initial clearance.

CRIMINAL RECORD CLEARANCE

When an individual receives a criminal record clearance, he/she may work, reside or volunteer in a licensed facility. The clearance will remain active as long as the individual is associated to a licensed facility. If an individual is disassociated from a facility, he/she must be associated to another facility (or the same facility if they are rehired) within 2 years or he/she will become inactive. If an individual becomes inactive, he/she must be fingerprinted and cleared again before working, residing or volunteering in a licensed facility.

A newly printed individual's clearance will be listed on the California Background Clearance Listing found in the website known as (Http://ccld.ca.gov/docs/dojclear/) for 30 days. A licensee may verify clearances older than 30 days by calling their local CCLD Regional Office.

Transferring a Clearance

Active criminal record clearances may be transferred from one state licensed facility to another by a license applicant or licensee. Clearances may not be transferred from a state licensed facility to a county licensed facility or from county to state. If an individual has an <u>active clearance, he/she shall not be re-fingerprinted again.</u> Licensees or license applicants may contact their local CCLD Regional Office to verify the individual's status.

To request a clearance transfer, a licensee or license applicant must submit an LIC. 9182, Criminal Record Clearance Transfer Request form (http://www.dss.cahwnet.gov/pdf/ LIC. 9182 PDF) to their local CCLD Regional Office. Transfers to more than one facility may be requested on one form. If needed, attach a list of each facility number to which the individual is to be transferred.

All clearance transfer requests must be submitted to the Department before the individual, (who is subject to the transfer) has client contact with the residents or the licensee will be in violation of the law and subject to a $100 civil penalty.

CRIMINAL RECORD EXEMPTIONS

When an applicant or licensee receives an exemption notification letter from CBCB concerning an employee, volunteer or adult resident, he/she must decide whether to request the exemption for that individual. If an exemption is desired, the licensee must assist the individual by mailing all exemption documentation to CBCB. If the licensee does not wish to pursue the exemption, and subsequently terminates the employee or removes him/her from the residency, the licensee must give that person the "Individual Exemption Request" included with the notification letter. This document allows the individual to request an exemption on his/her own behalf. A person seeking an individual exemption may not be present in any community care facility until an exemption is granted by CBCB.

Prospective foster parents applying for certification through a foster family agency may not seek an individual exemption. The foster family agency must decide if an exemption is desired. However, employees of a foster family agency can seek an individual exemption.

What Convictions Require Exemption?

All convictions other than minor traffic violations, including misdemeanors, felonies and convictions that occurred a long time ago shall require an exemption. However, individuals convicted of serious crimes such as robbery, sexual battery, child abuse, elder or dependant adult abuse, rape, arson or kidnapping are not eligible for an exemption as they are not qualified.

The Department of Social Services is prohibited by law from granting exemptions to individuals convicted of certain crimes. For a complete list of crimes for which the Department is prohibited from granting an exemption you may contact your local Community Care Licensing office.

To request an exemption the following items must be submitted:

1. A written request from the licensee/applicant on behalf of the individual.

2. A detailed description of the individual's responsibilities and roles at the facility.

3. A written request from the affected individual on his/her own behalf if the licensee chooses not to request an exemption and a termination of the individual from employment because of the individual's criminal history.

4. A copy of the signed Criminal Record Statement (LIC. 508) that was completed at the time of hire.

5. A written statement signed by the individual describing the events surrounding each conviction including the approximate date, what happened, why it happened, and any other information he/she deem important to understand the incident/crime. The individual shall also address what he/she has done or how his/her life has changed to prevent him/her from committing this type of offense again.

6. Documentation (Minute Order, court ordered Judgment of Conviction or a letter from the Probation Officer) that the individual's current or last period of probation (optional).

7. Written verification of any training, classes, courses, rehabilitation treatment / counseling sessions completed.

8. Three signed character reference statements including the telephone number and address of the person writing the reference. Character references must be current and may not be from the individual's relatives or family members nor from employees associated with the licensed facility. The character reference letters must be dated. References must be on a reference statement form (LIC. 301E).

9. The individual's current mailing address and telephone number.

10   A copy of all police reports involving the crime(s) for which the individual was convicted, or a letter from law enforcement stating that a report no longer exists.

Deadline for Exemptions

All requested exemption documents must be received by CBCB no later than 45 days from the date of the exemption notification letter. If documentation is not received by the deadline, the case will be closed. If an exemption is requested, it will take at least 75 days to process. The applicant or licensee seeking the exemption will be notified in writing of CBCB's decision. With individual exemption requests, the individual seeking the exemption will be notified.

Right to Appeal

If a request for exemption is denied, the individual may file for an appeal in writing. The appeal must be received by the Department of Social Services no later than 15 days from the date of the denial notification letter. Appeals received after the deadline will not be considered.

Get Fingerprinted thru Live-Scan.

No one is allowed in a residential care facility and to have initial contact with the residents without first being fingerprinted and cleared prior to reporting for work or duty.

One of the basic requirements in becoming a Facility Administrator is to be fingerprinted through Live-Scan. Years ago, the practice back then was fingerprinting thru the local police department. But there were so much problems with that practice as it took a little while (at least four to six months) before an individual is determined to be clear of any criminal records. By that time, that individual have already caused problems or perhaps he/she already quit and finds another job or worse could hurt the residents. With the advent of technology, we now have the capability to learn about an individual's history in just seconds with the help of a computer database that is connected to various government agencies such as the FBI and the DOJ that gives us a more accurate and reliable information in just a very short time. Live-Scan is a private company vendorized by the state to provide fingerprinting services to most agencies and entities recognized by the Department of Social Services and DDS, Health Care Licensing etc... Live-Scan has a computer access to the database of the Department of Justice and the Federal Bureau of Investigation to verify if a given fingerprint belongs to an individual with civil and criminal records of any sort or degree.

Fingerprinting process takes a few minutes and a verification that the agency is informed that a particular individual is applying for a job as a care-provider or as a service provider is cleared within same day. If the individual has pending criminal investigation or record, he/she is notified as well as the employer or the local public agency. As soon as a notification of an individual's status is received, as an employer, it is your responsibility to immediately inform the individual of the adverse information that you received and such individual must immediately be prevented from continuous contact with the residents in order to secure the safety and well-being of the residents/consumers.

The cost of the fingerprinting may vary from location and depending on the particular applied job or position. Contact your local Live Scan fingerprinting provider.

How does the fingerprinting process works?

The rolling of fingerprints using ink and a standard 8" X 8" fingerprint card is being replaced by Electronic fingerprinting technology. This technology electronically transfers images of fingerprints and personal information to the Department of Justice (DOJ) and the Federal Bureau of Investigations FBI in a matter of seconds, compared to how it was before when fingerprint cards had to be send through the U.S. mail. The results of the DOJ-FBI fingerprint check are sent to Community Care Licensing (CCL) for review and update.

The individual will be provided with an Applicant Submission form from CCL to fill out before having their fingerprints scanned. This form will also automatically request a Child Abuse Central Index (CACI) check if needed.

The following steps will help you understand the Live-Scan Fingerprint process.

1. You can obtain the Live Scan Application Submission form, information and updates from the local Community Care Licensing office (license provider) and through their website or from any CCL District Office. This form will take the place of a BID-7B fingerprint card when using the Live Scan process.

2. The individual fills out the form and calls the Live-Scan vendor at 1-800-315-4507 to schedule an appointment. At that time, the appointment scheduler will ask you to provide the information on the Applicant Submission form. An appointment schedule at any district office nearest you will be provided for your convenience. It is very important that you call within 24 hours to confirm or to cancel and reset an appointment if you are unable to attend the designated schedule.

3. When you come to the district office, the Live-Scan operator will already have your information in the computer. You will then have your fingerprints scanned by the operator.

4. The Live-Scan operator will then inform you of the charges, which include all necessary services DOJ, CACI, and FBI (CACI if applicable only) and the transmission of prints.

5. After recording the fingerprints and applicant information, the data will be electronically transmitted to DOJ for processing.

6. DOJ will send the results of the fingerprint check to CCL.

Secure CPR-First Aid Certification

To be able to serve in this type of facilities where the people you care for are very vulnerable to various elements relative to their care and well being, you must be able to secure CPR and First Aid certificate which may be acquired from the local community schools, colleges, American Red Cross, American Heart Association and other various entities and locations for a fee which may vary between $ 45.00 up to more than $85.00. The certificate is valid for one or two years depending on the agency providing the certification.

For Adult/Senior Facilities, Administrator must secure an eight (8) hour HIV- Hepatitis Certification Course.

Most facilities for children, adults senior residential care Facilities and day programs require their staff including administrators to undergo 8-hours of HIV-Hepatitis Certification prior to being employed in a facility. The classes may be offered in places and schools where classes such as CPR certification is provided.

Direct Support Professionals

Direct support professionals in Service Levels 2, 3, and 4 facilities employed before January 1, 2001 must satisfactorily complete the first 35-hour training segment (Year 1) by January 1, 2002; and satisfactorily complete the second 35-hour training segment (Year 2) by January 1, 2003.

Direct support professionals in Service Levels 2, 3, and 4 facilities employed on or after January 1, 2001, have one year from date of hire to satisfactorily complete the first 35-hour training segment; and, two years from the date of hire to complete the second 35-hour training segment. Recognizing that direct support professionals are a key to the provision of quality care, it is essential that they be trained and competent to meet the needs of individuals they serve. Towards this end, DDS has implemented a two-year, 70-hour standardized statewide competency-based training program which is mandatory for all CCF direct support professionals and CCF administrators who provide direct care. The 70 hours of training is divided into two equal parts of 35 hours each to be completed in successive years. Those required to take the training have the opportunity to take a challenge test for each of the 35-hour segments. Those who pass the challenge test for either of the 35-hour training segments will not be required to take that segment. Testing and training are based upon core competencies or skills necessary for satisfactory direct support professionals' job performance.

Direct Support Professional Training is provided by local Regional Occupational Centers and Programs (ROCPs) in their respective communities at no cost to enrollees. The ROCPs are using instructors who have practical work experience in the provision of services to people with developmental disabilities. To date, approximately 17,000 people have successfully completed the Year 1 training requirements. Both Year 1 and Year 2 training is now being offered by the ROCPs.

Chapter 5: THE BUSINESS PLAN

Step 3. Create a Business Plan

Preparing a business plan is the most important step that a beginner needs to do first before incurring any other unnecessary expenses in the business. To those who do not have any experience in setting up a business and are in it for the first time, it is extremely important to prepare a business plan first which also includes a marketing research on the business particularly client sources, income, start up expenses, long term and short term projections etc...

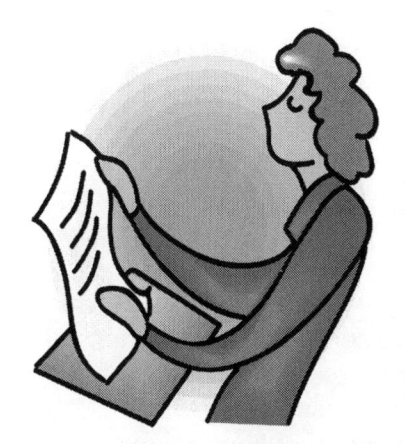

A business plan can be compared to a road map that draws possible path to either success or to failure. To those who do not consider failure as an option, creating a plan is very important. There are lot of books and computer software available in the local stores that you can find useful in preparing a business plan. Most of them are user friendly and easy to understand.

Below is a general outline of a typical business plan. This outline indicates the sample topics or items that the preparer may need to discuss in presenting the plan.

A Business Plan

    1.   Cover Sheet
    2.   Statement of purpose
    3.   Table of Contents

I. The Business

    A.   Description of the Business
    B.   Marketing
    C.   Competition

     D. Operating Procedures
     E. Personnel
     F. Financial Data

II. Financial Data

     A. Capital equipment and supply list
     B. Balance Sheet
     C. Break even analysis
     D. Pro-forma income projections (profit and loss statement)
     E. Three year summary Detail by month, first year Detail by quarter, second and third years. Assumption upon which projections were based from
     F. Pro-forma cash flow

III. Supporting Documents

     A. Tax returns for last three years
     B. Personal financial statement
     C. Resume of all professionals and their respective services
     D. Others

Based on the financial information presented on the business plan and after determination that the project is viable, the next thing to do is to determine its affordability in starting and maintaining the business. The applicant must provide proof of financial capacity as well as the ability to maintain the business in the long term. In line with this provision, Community Care Licensing (CCLD) will verify all pertinent financial information that the applicant will submit including financial statement, and verification of deposit from the bank. Typically, the agency needs to know if these start-up funds are readily available for the sole purpose of setting the business.

If you are to raise a question as to how much money you may need to prove your serious intent (as an applicant) in starting the business, there is no right or wrong answer. Generally, the amount of reserve in the applicant's bank statement intended for the business must at least be sufficient to cover daily operation of the business for at least three to six months with the assumption that the business is up and ready to accept clients at any short notice. There are a lot of ways to go about this requirement including the acquisition of a loan from local banks using equity on real estate property, IRA, 401K, 457, Savings Bonds, Mutual Funds, stocks, bonds etc... Also, try to consider creative financing by pulling in a business partner (s) or a group of professionals who are willing to invest their experience, time and money in the project.

A. THE START UP COST

Part of the requirements in the initial process is for the applicant to submit an operating budget proposal together with the application. The budget amount must coincide with the prepared business plan. This budget statement shall reflect the total amount of money that the Community Care Licensing Office will require to verify from the applicant's bank to show that the applicant is ready to do serious business.

Without this budget statement in the application and the bank verification, licensing may hold the application temporarily or may require it as part of the conditions for issuance of a temporary license. Included in this section is a sample budget statement for the reader to have an idea as to the format and the content of a budget proposal.

SAMPLE START UP COST

Application Cost	$ 200.00
Live-Scan Fingerprinting	$ 184.00
Administrative Certification Course	$ 440.00
Market Research and Consultation	$ 3,000.00
Administrator's Certificate	$ 100.00
Articles of Incorporation	$ 100.00
Gas /Mileage	$ 80.00
Law and Business Software	$ 80.00
Hep/HIV Certification	$ 100.00
Accounting Software	$ 80.00
Fictitious Business Name/	$ 80.00
City Registration	$ 65.00
Business Insurance/Site Deposit	$ 300.00
Automobile Insurance Deposit	$ 100.00
Professional/General Liability Insurance (Deposit)	$ 600.00
Workers Comp. Deposit	$ 800.00
Non-Hire Transport Insurance	$ 800.00
Van Lease deposit	$ 5,000.00
Others	$ 200.00

Office Cost

Computer	$ 1,000.00
Filing Cabinets	$ 200.00
Telephone-Fax	$ 150.00
10-Key calculator	$ 50.00
Answering machine	$ 40.00
Database	$ 65.00
Pens/pencils/Supplies	$ 100.00
Book Shelves	$ 300.00
Wall calendars/decorations	$ 65.00

Equipment and supplies cost

Tables and chairs	$ 500.00
Furniture	$ 1,500.00
Cooking supplies	$ 100.00
Art and Crafts	$ 300.00
Computers for consumer	$ 1,000.00
Cleaning supplies	$ 120.00
Supplies	$ 40.00
Sound system	$ 500.00
Games and Recreation	$ 300.00
Dishes/Utensils	$ 240.00
Pots and pans	$ 100.00
Medicine cabinet/storage	$ 60.00
Refrigerator	$ 500.00
Dishwasher	$ 500.00
Washer and Dryer	$ 700.00

Others $ 1,900.00

Total Start-Up Cost :
Excluding Fixed and Variable Cost   **($ 22,199.00)**

3 months Cash Reserve
Requirement   **($ 66,597.00)**

As per Licensing and Regional Center requirement, this amount must reflect in the bank statement and must state that the fund intended is solely for the use of the business.

It is always a good business practice to have sufficient amount of cash reserves to get by while waiting for your first residents. It is also recommend for all start ups to extend their cash reserves up to six month in case the process takes longer than expected or to come up with some sort of creative financing or perhaps resort to creative spending. While waiting for the first referral clients, it is a good idea that the administrator should be able to literally flex his/her role in order to be able to stretch the cash reserves to the conservative limit. There is no proven prediction as to how soon will the facility receive its first clients. There are some who had the experience where it took them at least one year before they received their first client. With this in mind, it is a must for the business operator not to quit his/her day jobs yet until the revenues become stable. That is why business planning is very important.

The next challenge that you will need to face is the issue of whether it is practical to buy an already existing business or to start from the scratch? Well, if you want to know more about this, read on because this book will be discussing the practical side of purchasing an already existing business.

NO CASH RESERVES AVAILABLE YET?

When you figure out after drawing your business plan and get the shock of your life as you find out that the business could require more money than you expected... suddenly you said "yikes, I do not have that amount of money right now". Well, there is another alternative besides coming up with your own personal funds. Why not ask for "free money". Yes! Free money can come in a form of "request for a grant" from a non-profit foundation/organization or companies or a public entity that will loan you the money that you need or match your available funds "dollar for dollar" based on what-ever amount you can afford to pitch in. This subject will be discussed later on in the next chapter on "FREE MONEY: WHERE TO SECURE FINANCING, WHERE TO GET FREE MONEY, GRANTS, DONATIONS, GIFTS ETC.. TO FINANCE THE BUSINESS". There will also be discussions on other alternate sources that you might want to consider in securing funding for your business.

On the topic of securing funding for your business, this book will describe to you a variety of ways and resources to get funding including the citation of several names of companies and agencies that you can solicit from. The best part of it, is that most of these companies may not even require you to pay them back, *as sometimes the LOAN/GRANT could be FREE.*

Too good to be true? Read on and find out more in the next chapter.

Chapter 6 : FINANCING THE BUSINESS

A. FREE MONEY: WHERE TO SECURE FINANCING, FREE MONEY, GRANTS, GIFTS DONATIONS, ETC... TO FINANCE THE BUSINESS

Secure Financing for the Business

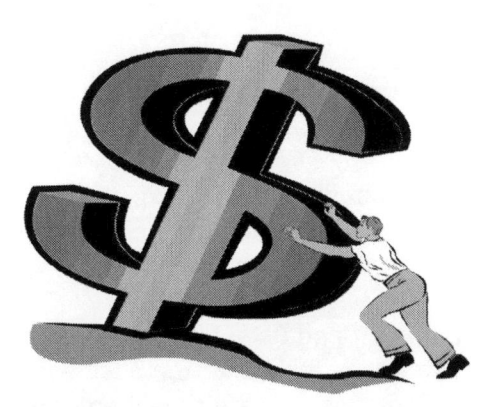

After making financial decision based on the feasibility of the business plan you made, the next move would be to figure out whether to continue on to the next level. Should you decide that this is not the right business for you, at least your over all cost is still very minimal, which is just the cost of this book and a little bit of your leisure time. However, if the decision is to move on forward to the next level, the dilemma would then be to figure out where to get funding necessary to get the business started. This section is written to help you answer a lot of the questions that you might have concerning the challenges you encounter when setting up this business. The ideas that you are about to learn here are not guaranteed 100% effective as results may vary depending on individual situations, availability of the program at the time of request, state funding etc... Nevertheless, continue with your reading and try to find out what applies to your particular situation or at least explore the possibilities of funding your business.

Finding a start up capital is never easy. Even if you have an excellent business idea but do not have sufficient collateral to back it up, it will be very tough most particularly if you do not know what to do and where to go. It is not impossible to find available resources out there. It is just a matter of finding out where to start. Undoubtedly, perseverance and commitment to your business idea will serve as an important key in unlocking the potentials to these challenges that you initially face. Do not be discouraged. As told several times by famous author Napoleon Hill in his book, "Think and Grow Rich" where he described successful people like Thomas Edison, Andrew Carnegie, Henry Ford... he said... "all achievement, all earned riches, have their beginnings in an idea." It is up to you to make that idea a reality. You have full control. As Sir Winston Churchill of England once said in his speech after the war ..."Never, Never, Never, Never Ever Give Up".

Are you looking for a way to buy a home or to fund your new business ?

There are quite a number of creative ways to buy a home and in turn converting that home for use as your business. Listed in this chapter are ways to do it which shall also be discussed in the succeeding chapters. By the way, when you are in business, your expenses in maintaining the home-office is also tax deductible. (Consult with your accountant on this subject)

Here is a list of resources that you might find useful in your search to finance your business or buying a house to use for the business. Be advised that the organizations cited may have their requirements and guidelines that you have to observe in order for them to consider your proposal.

For funding alternatives, consider the following options:

1. **Personal funds, money from friends and relatives, get a business partner, look for an investor:**

When it comes to financing your own business, the first thing that you as a start-up need to look into is your personal finance, how much money you have saved or is expecting to receive while getting this business started. Perhaps you might want to check your savings, income from your jobs, retirement funds, IRA, stock and bonds or even inheritance from a long lost uncle etc... You must remember that you need to have at least three months of cash reserves to stay afloat in the business and in worse scenario, need to learn how to stretch your money for up to six months or until you receive your first client. To some, it took them longer than a year to get their first service. So, be ready financially, mentally and psychologically.

2. **Regional Centers, Probation, Dept. of Aging and other Placement Agencies:**

Another resources to consider are your local placement agencies, Regional Centers, Dept. of Children and family Services DCFS, Child Protective Services CPS, Dept. of Aging, Dept. of Corrections and Probation in your local area as they may serve as a starting point for reference and advice concerning financing and pertinent information on the available services. Most if not all of them offer **Request For Proposals RFP's** from time to time depending on the need for a given service (as discussed on the topic of **RFPs'**). If caring for the disabled population is your focus, you might want to consult with your local Regional Centers for start-up funding. There are 21 Regional Centers in the state of California and they all (if not most of them) have budget allocations for start-up businesses like yours depending on the type of services they are considering to finance. Depending on the county and available state funds allocated for a given service need, Regional Centers are excellent source for start-up capital funds. They provide grants or loans for certain "much needed services or priority projects" and sometimes if the grantee stays in excellent standing and meets the standard of expectations specified on the provider's service contract for at least three years from start of the business, **the grants/loans given may be waived which means that the recipient may not need to pay it back therefore it is FREE.** There are a number of Regional Centers that provides funding allocations for start-up capital up to more than $50,000.00 to qualified vendors. To find out more information, contact the Resource Unit and Vendorization Unit at any Regional Center office.

3. **US Small Business Administration (SBA).**

SBA is the largest source of long-term small business financing in the nation. Many start-up individuals have used SBA loans to start or expand businesses that operate from a licensed small 6-bed facility such as group homes and board and care homes to a medium size facility including intermediate care facilities for the developmentally disabled. In order to be eligible for a loan, a business must be operated for profit and qualify as a small business under the SBA size standard criteria:

a. Use of proceeds: The loan proceeds may be used for a variety of business purposes including working capital, inventory, machinery and equipment, leasehold improvements and the acquisition of business property.

b. Loan term: The maturity of the loan is dependent on the use of the loan proceed and varies from five to seven years for working capital, ten years for fixed assets or 25 years for real estate acquisitions.

c. Interest rates: The interest rates are variable and are negotiated between the lender (the bank) and the borrower; however, the lenders generally may not charge more than prime rate. The individual can approach a local bank that provides SBA loans and the SBA shall guarantee the payment of the loan when due.

d. Collateral: SBA requires that sufficient assets be pledged as collateral for the loan to ensure that the business owner has a substantial interest in the success of the business. Although SBA will not decline a loan application due to lack of collateral, lenders will require a reasonable amount to provide a secondary source of repayment.

SBA will help you obtain conventional financing through loan guarantees or loans made by private lenders. To cite a few sample available programs:

1. Small loan guarantees
2. Seasonal line of credit guarantees
3. Handicapped assistance loans
4. Venture capital
5. Loans for disabled and Vietnam Veterans
6. Long term loans

In addition to these programs, SBA offers training, technical help and counseling with three partner organizations namely:

- Service Corps of retired Executives (SCORE) that provides free training and one-on-one counseling from volunteers.

- Small Business Development Centers (SBDC's) providing training, research, counseling and other kinds of assistance.
- Small Business Institutes providing free management studies provided by business students under faculty directions at more than 500 universities.

4 Fannie Mae:

Responding to a growing need for group housing for the developmentally disabled individuals, the company introduced Community Living which is a $10 Billion Dollar affordable housing initiative, purchases qualifying mortgages made by Fannie Mae approved lenders to individuals for profit corporations and government agencies. Properties eligible for purchases under community living program are one or two unit dwellings that are permanent group residences for developmentally disabled individuals in the community. Please call your local Fannie Mae Lender on this program.

5. **US Department of Housing and Urban Development (HUD): US Dept. of HUD, has various programs that the reader might want to explore.**

    (a). **Title 1 Housing and Community Development Act of 1974**
    known as Community Development Block Grants: Entitlement for communities to carry out a wide range of community development activities directed towards neighborhood revitalization, economic development and improved community facilities and services.

    (b). **Community Development Block Grants:**
    (Non-Entitlement) for States and Small Cities: Federal Aid to promote sound community development primarily for the benefit of individuals with low and moderate income. The applicant must give maximum feasible priority to activities and services that will benefit the low to moderate income population in the community.

- **(c). HOPE for Homeownership of Single Family Homes:**
  A national program offering homeownership opportunities to lower income families and individuals by providing federal assistance to finance eligible homebuyer's direct purchase and rehabilitation of eligible family properties. The program may also be used for the acquisition and rehabilitation of single family properties for sale and occupancy by families at affordable prices.

- **(d). Shelter Plus (S+C):**
  Grants for rental assistance in combination with support services to the homeless persons with disabilities.

- **(e). Supportive Housing for Persons with Disabilities:**
  Section 811 Cranston-Gonzales National Affordable Housing Act where assistance is provided as capital advances to finance construction, rehabilitation or acquisition of structures to develop a range of housing options for the developmentally disabled individuals in the community. (Funding for this program is dependent on the Notice of Funding Availability). This program is intended for developing housing options ranging from group homes to dwelling units with multi-family housing, cooperatives or condominiums. It works by providing capital advance and rental assistance to a project. The organization eligible for funding under this program are non-profits only where the funds can be used for construction, rehabilitation or acquisition of group homes.

- **(f). Department of Housing & Community Development:**
  This organization have community programs geared towards the improvement and development of the community particularly affordable housing or cooperative housing for low income families.

  a. California Indian Assistance Program (CIAP)
  b. California Housing Rehabilitation Program
  c. Family Housing Demonstration Program
  d. Farm worker Housing Grant Program
  e. Federal Emergency Shelter Grant Program
  f. Home Investment Partnership Program

g. Permanent Housing for the Handicapped Homeless

(g). PRIVATE PHILATROPIC FOUNDATIONS:
The following are some list of foundations that provides grants geared towards assisting the needs of the developmentally disabled which means that the non-profit organization may seek assistance in the establishment of the business. The information on these organizations may be found thru the world wide web.

1. The Ahmanson Foundation
2. BankAmerica Foundation
3. California Community Foundation
4. SH Cowell Foundation
5. Wallace Alexander Gerbode Foundation
6. William and Flora Hewlett Foundation
7. The Henry J. Kaiser Family Foundation
8. Walter S. Johnson Foundation
9. W.M. Keck Foundation
10. Wilbur D. May Foundation
11. The David and Lucille Packard Foundation
12. Milken Family Medical Foundation
13. Weingart Foundation

WRITING A GRANT PROPOSAL

In requesting for financial support or a grant, the reader is advised to research on how to prepare a grant request. There are a lot of books available at the book stores and computer software shops on writing grants. (A suggested sample format in this book is also included). As you read through the subject, you may come up with your own format depending on the project, company or entity that the grant is intended for, the purpose and of course the mission /objective. For foundations or corporations, in order to apply for a grant the writer should always prepare a cover letter describing who he/she is, briefly discuss the plan and specify the amount and purpose of funding being requested. Try to limit the proposal letter to about three pages of narrative and must be signed by the Executive Officer. It is also a wise idea to attach a copy of your company's annual budget for the past year and an audited financial statement, an IRS letter of Determination (Non-Profit), a letter of support and an annual report if you have. Otherwise, a cover letter and a business plan/grant proposal will be sufficient.

Preparing a grant is somewhat similar to a business plan as it indicates the amount of money needed and for what purpose. Included in this section is a Summary Draft of a Grant and what a grant proposal should contain.

Components of a Proposal/ GRANT

I. Summary
II. Introduction
III. Problem Statement
IV. Objectives
V. Methods
VI. Evaluation
VII. Future or other necessary funding
VIII Proposal Budget Estimates
IX. Time Chart

Tips in writing a Grant Proposal:

1. Include a cover letter

2. Be brief and positive

3. Avoid unsupported assumptions

4. It must be written in clean, neat paper and must be in English.

5. Write to an organization that supports your objectives and mission statement.

6. You may use the same budget estimates that you will submit to Community Care Licensing.

An Easy Guide On How to Establish Your First Residential Care Facility

7.   Provide a Business Plan

8.   Good luck and be positive.

BUY A HOUSE WITH LITTLE DOWN OR USING CREATIVE FINANCING?

This topic is further discussed in Chapter 9: ACQUIRE THE PROPERTY/BUSINESS. As the old saying …"if the deal sounds too good to be true chances are….. Well, just be very careful. There are hundreds of self-help books available out there and tons of info-commercials seen on television every late night selling ideas on how to buy a house or a property with little or no money down. A lot of those deals are real and there are quite a few that are doubtful so, it is purely up to your common sense to decide which one to choose.

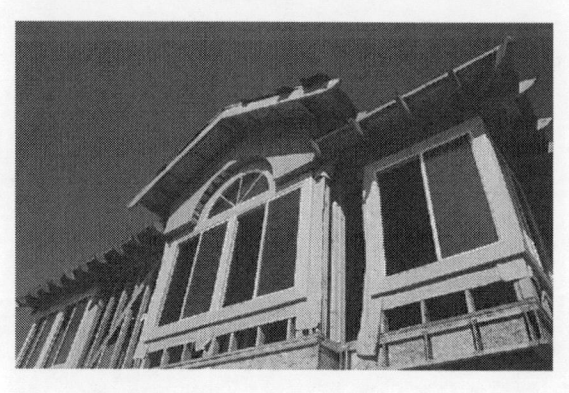

There are also programs for veterans and low income individuals as well as for the disabled. There are a few suggestions to observe for those who might want to consider this approach: Stick to the basics which is save your hard earned cash wisely, maintain good credit standing, look for a property that you like to live in or you can afford to fix conservatively, deal with a seller who is willing to make the deal work for both of you on a win-win situation, work out a good price and end up with the best financing package that suits you on a long or short term plan. Attend auctions, foreclosure sales (ie: VA Foreclosures) and bid on a property you like based on comparables or feasible price that you are willing to pay for. The highest bidder wins, so how high you are willing to risk is purely up to you. Look at a deal with the lowest cash investment requirement, figure out your high and your low bidding price. Chances are, you will not get all the properties you want but at least get the one that you are happy with as far as future earning is concerned.

Get the right financing by dealing with an experienced real estate finance consultant and plan what you intend to do with the property while you are waiting for the Program Design to be approved.

PROGRAM STATEMENT
Chapter 7: PROGRAM DESIGN

Step 4: Prepare a Draft of the Program Design

The next step that you are about to go through can either be done between the Step 1 and Step 8 preferably after attending the Initial Facility Administrator Certification Course where in most cases the topics on the subject of drawing a program design is discussed. By taking the Initial Administrator Certification Course, most course providers will help you learn the basics on facility management which also includes your understanding of the business in particular. Once you understand what the business is all about, then you can technically draw your own program design based on what you learned from your training.

In order to be able to draw a program statement/design, you will need to have a clear understanding of Title 22 and Title 17, that which basically regulates and provides guidelines for all residential care facilities. You will also need to consult with your licensing program analyst and to secure a copy of an "Application for a License to Operate a Residential Care Facility" in which you need to specify what type of facility you are applying for.

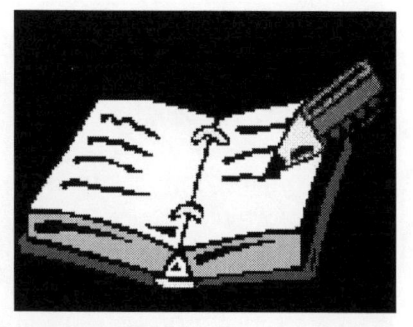

For group Homes, there is a blue covered application packet complete with the forms you will need in applying for a license. In the case of other types of facilities, you can down load from the Department of Social Services website under applications and forms that contain a print out of a complete application packet that you need to complete in drawing a program design. The application is very simple and easy to understand.

Most of the time, the applicant is confused because he/she does not know exactly what type of facility he/she is considering and what other important things to write about in the program design. Well, I have some good news for you. **To be able to help you in this confusing procedure, included in this reading material are**

sample program designs that I personally wrote and are found in Exhibit Two and Three which you might want to use as a guide in drawing your own program design.

To those who are new in the business, you might want to ask your self how do you go about designing an operating manual for a business that you do not know much about. This is one of the most difficult challenge that you as a beginner will encounter when you start the business. For some of you who may have experience in the business, but as a staff or administrator, your role in your job is limited to the generalized operation of the business and not on the over-all extensive and meticulous part of the business. Performing the role of a staff is one thing but writing the program design on the matter is totally different from what you think it is.

In writing a program design, the applicant must take into consideration the information described in the application. For instance, you are considering serving needs of the elderly population and most elderly people are possibly non-ambulatory, therefore on the program design, you need to describe the home/facility to suit the needs of the elderly, or the disabled perhaps you might need to retrofit the home based on the standards that will accommodate non-ambulatory residents which requires safety equipment, handle bars on the walk ways, in the bathrooms etc.. The application must reflect the items specified in the program design therefore, it is advisable to initially draft a program design and then fill in the application information based on what appears on the program design.

When filling the application, you need to practice writing your answers on a photocopy and then eventually typing or neatly hand write the answer on the original application form.

When you are not comfortable drawing your own program design, you might have two options:

Two options:

First option is to contract the service of an experienced consultant who will prepare and draw the program design just for your specification for a fee that typically costs starting at $2,500.00 up to $10,000.00 per program design depending factors such as type of facility, the level of care proposed and the extensive work that is required specially when frequent correction and modifications of the design is observed.

Your second option is to draw the program design your self. With the help of the sample program designs that is included in this book **(Exhibit Two and Three: Sample Program Designs)**, you are literally saving yourself time and money perhaps over $5,000.00 to $10,000.00 in consultation fee. Honestly speaking, it is difficult to draw a program design especially if you do not know what you are doing and do not know exactly what to write about. The sample program designs that are included in this book will make it convenient for you when you draw your own program design. It could be a very tedious and meticulous undertaking but it is well worth a try. If you have the patience and the resourcefulness to research on the subjects you want to cover in your design, you will do great. As a matter of fact, most (if not all) of my former students who graduated from the Initial Administrator Certification Courses that I taught in the past started their business and wrote their own program designs themselves. They all did well and so can you. Do not worry so much about how the design will be. The Program Analyst assigned to help you will guide you accordingly. As soon as you submit the design, a designated LPA will coordinate with you within 90 days from date of receipt to discuss your program and a correction plan on your design will be made for you to revise your program. Some requirements may not be that significant that your LPA have the option to grant you a provisional license with conditions subject to your completion of the missing requirement.

As you are responsible for drawing your own program design, you need to come up with creative ideas possibly from my sample design. There is no need in making major deviation from the sample as long as it serves your purpose in the design. Picture for yourself some of the things you want to implement in your facility then put in simple words and describe how those ideas will benefit the consumers/clients. If you need to write the idea in a step-by-step process, it is also acceptable. You can use my ideas and then modify them according to your specifications. WARNING: The Community Care Licensing office may be aware of this sample design that I wrote for hundreds of my readers like you, so, to avoid possible rejection of your program design, it is very wise for you to just get the idea and come up with your own style. **(Please refer to Exhibit Two and Three: Sample Program Designs).**

In order to write a good program design, it is always best to draw a draft and correct it as you deem fit. When you write your draft, show it to a friend or to someone who has experience in the business. It is always expected for a program design draft to be revised more than three times or as often as necessary. Do not worry too much about how your program will look or sound like. Write it down and submit it as soon as you are ready. The design is subject for review and subsequent revisions anyway. Consult with your LPA analyst if there are things that you will find unclear about your program design.

Here is a general guideline on what you need to know when you write your program design.

WHAT IS A PROGRAM DESIGN ?

A program design is defined as a collection of illustrations narrated in written format describing unique combination of services proposed to be observed in a given type of setting or facility to meet the needs and services of given consumers/clients that the applicant wants to serve. It is a written description of how a facility will function in order to satisfy the needs and services of the people living within the facility. In order for a home or a facility to be granted a license, it must present a program design which reflect the promises and intentions of the facility as to how they will accomplish their objectives of meeting the needs of the people who will be entrusted to live and benefit from the facility. A facility program design may be unique in its own style or service format depending on the type of consumers it aims to serve. Every residential care facility must be licensed and have a designated level or rate established in order to accept placements from the Regional Centers, Dept. of Mental Health, County Social Services or Probation Departments.

Although there is no standard format for a program design, the unique part of it is for the writer or creator of the program design to use his/her creativity and resourcefulness in converting applicable regulations into a narrative writing to illustrate how the facility will care for the individuals who will be placed in the facility. The program design may be subjected to revisions and corrections (pending review of the application for a license) by the designated licensing program analyst until the description is acceptable based on given standards set by the regulation in order for the facility to be issued a license to operate a facility.

In order to have a better idea of how a program design will be established, here are suggested contents and topics to be discussed thoroughly in a typical program design:

Contents of a Program Design

a. Mission Statement
b. Objective
c. Company Description
d. Organization
e. Organizational Chart
f. Staffing and Administration
g. Policies and procedures
h. Emergency plan
i. Intervention and therapy
j. Type of Facility
k. Location
l. Consumer Characteristics
m. Statement of Purpose
n. Services Offered and its Delivery System
o. Activities
p. Menu
q. Schedules of Activities
r. Staffing Plan and Schedules
t. Consumer Assessment and Evaluations
u. Continuum of Care

All residential care facilities including foster family homes, small family homes, group homes, residential care for adults, the elderly, the chronically ill; day programs and transition homes share similarities in application requirements and procedures. Program designs may also bear common general resemblance but due to the nature of their specific services and level requirements, it may show a small deviation but the over-all approach may be similar. Regardless of what type of facility that you are contemplating in establishing (foster homes, day care center, residential care facility for children-adults or seniors), this book will be very useful to you in many ways particularly in preparing for a program design.

For the purpose of simplifying the discussion on the subject of submitting a program design, this book shall use for illustration the process used in submitting a group home statement/application. The reason for being is that the application process in a group home is extensive and covers considerable amount of subject matter broad enough to be used in applications for all other types of residential care facilities except for a few minor differences.

PROCESS FOR SUBMISSION OF INITIAL PROGRAM STATEMENT

First, complete the program statement/program design. Then, submit one copy of the program design to the host county (social services, city engineer's office, planning council, probation department, community care licensing, regional centers) and request for a letter of support. For new facilities in a local area, it is a good idea to provide a copy of your program design to the city council if in case the city has any questions or objections in giving you a business license to operate a facility in their city.

The host county reviews the program as described in the Program Statement and may schedule an interview and/or site visit to determine if the facility meets its needs. The host county must issue a letter of support before the next step is undertaken.

Secondly, submit three copies of the Program Statement and the county letter of support to the Community Care Licensing CCL District Office. (The support letter is not always a requirement for licensure.) In the case of group homes and other residential care facilities, the CCL District Office sends a copy of the Program Statement and the county letter of support to the Foster Care Rates Bureau or to the Dept. of Social Services, Community Care Licensing or Health Care Licensing in charge of issuing the License to Operate a Facility.

FORMAT FOR SUBMITING PROGRAM STATEMENT

All residential care facilities will be required to submit a program statement that contains the following format.

(1). Type or print clearly.

(2). Complete PART I PROGRAM IDENTIFICATION and PART II PROGRAM POPULATION, SERVICES AND CAPABILITIES.

(3). Prepare and compile the information and documentation requirement in PART III. PROGRAM NARRATIVE.

(4). Use the Table of Contents page included in the forms packet as the Table of Contents for your Program Statement.

(5). Number tabbed dividers or sheets to correspond to the numbers in the Table of Contents column entitled "Section Numbers". Place all appropriate materials behind each tabbed divider.

(6). Place all materials, in the order shown, in a three ring binder or folder. Place the Table of Contents in the front.

(7). Make three sets of copies a keep a copy for your records.

(When submitting revisions)

(8). Complete a new Part I PROGRAM IDENTIFICATION.

(9). Complete a revised Table of Contents; enter the date of the revision(s) in the "Date Revised" column opposite the section being revised.

(10). Clearly number and identify the revised material (or it will be returned to you).

(11). Keep a copy for your records.

Once the program design is reviewed, it is subject for revision or modification in accordance with the regulation. When the program appears adequate, and that all the described documentations are in order including a certificate of capacity and occupancy from the Fire Marshall, the home is subject to an initial visit to conduct a visual inspection of the facility and its physical location. Once the facility is certified to meet the regulatory standard, the home and its application may be ready for final review. In the case of other types of facilities, there are instance where the facility owner may be required to appear before the city council to seek a host letter or a resolution approving the establishment and operation of a facility in the area. The reason for this is that, most cities will be affected by your new business as far as safety, traffic and health is concerned. It is also a good idea for the applicant to introduce yourself to the neighborhood and let them know what your business is all about and discuss possible impact in the community.

For group homes, the applicant must submit revisions to the group home program statement when any changes are made to the program that could affect the license and/or the AFDC-FC rate. It is only necessary to submit the documents/pages that are revised, including a new Part I and revised Table of Contents.

It is not necessary to submit a complete new program statement. Changes to the group home program that are more than one Rate Classification Level (RCL) greater than the original RCL determination, i.e., new programs or program changes, must be submitted to and supported by the host county. This practice is also observed in other types of facilities when submitting a statement revision.

All revisions to the Program Design must be sent to the CCL District Office. Only the required revision must be resubmitted and not the whole program design that was originally sent. In the case of other facilities, the program statement shall remain under the review and evaluation of the licensing agency responsible for issuing the license.

Submit two copies of the revisions, and the host county letter of support if needed, to the CCL District Office. (The support letter is not a requirement for licensure.) The CCL District Office sends a copy of the revisions and the host county letter of support to the Foster Care Rates Bureau. In the case of other facility types, CCL will review the design and will make a final determination within 90 days. In the case of other facilities, the review and approval shall remain with the licensing agency responsible for the issuance of the license to operate a facility.

Chapter 8: THE BUSINESS ENTITY

Step 5: Establish your Business Entity

Sole Proprietorship, Corporation (For profit or Non- Profit), Partnership, Limited Liability Corporation

This is probably one of the biggest challenges for most start- ups unless you have legal background. Since you are not here to learn business law, the discussion on this subject will be limited to a simplified form. The goal is to give you, the reader general idea on the different types of business entities that are available and it is up to you to make your choice that you deem appropriate for your purpose. However, it is your responsibility to research on other information that is available to you and to make your own personal decision and of course to seek legal advice on the matter that you are getting into. There are useful books and reference materials available in the library and at a local bookstore on the subject of establishing a business and one of the major topics include corporations. It is very important to know what type of entity that you are interested in, to have the business name and entity registered with the Secretary of State in the state or county where the business will be established or located. For California residents you may check out the California Secretary of State website at: http://www.ss.ca.gov/ under Business Filings.

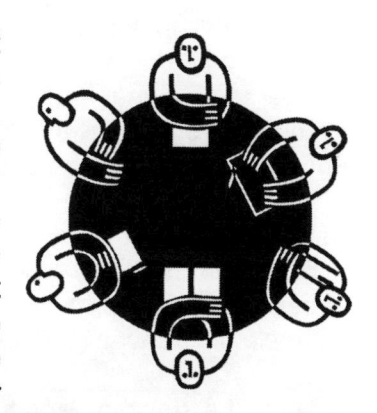

Generally, in establishing a residential care business, you have choices of any type of business entity: corporation, partnership, sole proprietorship, limited liability corporation LLC. The only exception to the general rule applies to Group Homes where it is required that all group homes for high risk children be limited to one choice of business entity which is to be a NON-PROFIT CORPORATION only. (In other states, the regulation on group homes may be different).
Corporations Compared to Sole Proprietorships and Partnerships

Corporations enjoy many advantages over partnerships and sole proprietorships. However, there are also disadvantages.

Advantages:

Stockholders are not liable for corporate debts. This is the most important aspect of a corporation. In a sole proprietorship and partnership, the owners are personally responsible for the debts of the business. In situations when the assets that belong to the sole proprietorship or partnership cannot satisfy the debt, creditors can go after each owner's personal bank account, house, etc. to make up the difference. On the other hand, if a corporation runs out of funds, its owners are usually off the hook.

Please note that under certain circumstances, an individual stockholder may be held liable for corporate debts. This is sometimes referred to as "piercing the corporate veil." Some of these circumstances include:

- If a stockholder personally guarantees a debt.
- If personal funds are intermingled with corporate funds.
- If a corporation fails to have director and shareholder meetings.
- If the corporation has minimal capitalization or minimal insurance.
- If the corporation fails to pay state taxes or otherwise violates state law.

Self-Employment Tax Savings. Earnings from a sole proprietorship are subject to self-employment taxes. Under corporation, only salaries (and not profits) are subject to such taxes. This advantage is most significant for stockholder-employees who take a salary of less than $72,600.

For example, if a sole proprietorship earns $60,000, tax would have to be paid on the entire $60,000. Assume that a corporation also earns $60,000 but $40,000 of that amount is paid in salary, and $20,000 is deemed as profit. In this case, the self-employment tax would not be paid on the $20,000 profit. This saves the stockholder-employee over $3,000 per year. Please note, however, that you should pay yourself a reasonable salary. The IRS frowns upon stockholder-employees who pay themselves too little.

Continuous life. The life of a corporation, unlike that of a partnership or sole proprietorship, does not expire upon the death of its stockholders, directors or officers of the corporation.

Easier to raise money. A corporation has many avenues to raise capital. It can sell shares of stock, and it can create new types of stocks, such as preferred stock, with different voting or profit characteristics. Most of all, investors can rest assured that they will not be personally liable for corporate debts.

Ease of transfer. Ownership interest in a corporation may be sold to third parties without disturbing the continued operation of the business. The business of a sole proprietorship or partnership, on the other hand, cannot be sold whole; instead, each of its assets, licenses and permits must be individually transferred, and new bank accounts and tax identification numbers are required.

Disadvantages

Higher cost. Corporations cost more to set up and to run than a sole proprietorship or partnership. For example, there are the initial formation fees, filing fees and annual state fees. These costs are partially offset by lower insurance costs.

Formal organization and corporate formalities. A corporation can only be created by filing legal documents with the state. In addition, a corporation must adhere to technical formalities which include holding director and shareholder meetings, recording minutes, having the board of directors approve major business transactions and corporate record-keeping. If these identified formalities are not kept accordingly, the stockholders risk losing their personal liability protection. While keeping corporate formalities is not difficult, it can be time-consuming. On the other hand, a sole proprietorship or partnership can commence and operate without any formal organizing or operating procedures not even a handwritten agreement.

Unemployment tax. A stockholder-employee of a corporation is required to pay unemployment insurance taxes on his or her salary, whereas a sole proprietor or partner is not.

In establishing a residential care business in general, there is no particular requirement as far as what type of entity one should have. *However, (as of the time this book is printed) in the case of the group home business, it is specifically required that a facility must be organized and operated by a non-profit corporation duly registered with the Secretary of State where the corporation is established.* Why does it have to be non-profit corporation? One reason is that, this requirement was specifically intended and is established by the Foster Care Rates Bureau with the opinion on the moral issue that people should not profit from displaced children. Some of the benefits of being non-profit include the entity's accessibility to grants, donations and gifts that are tax deductible, big earners needed to find a means to write off their excess earnings by donating their discretionary funds. In some states in the US, requirements may differ, so you are advised to consult with your local agency with regard to this requirement. For purposes of simplifying the discussion and instead of overloading you with information, the discussion will be limited on the subject of non-profit organization which basically gives the reader a simplified idea on what business entity to consider when establishing the business.

Most of the children placed in group homes are supported and funded by the Foster Care Rates Bureau (FCRB), under the coordination and supervision of the Department of Health and Human Services therefore it is important for a corporation to be non-profit in order to receive payments from the FCRB.

What is a non-profit corporation and how is it formed?

A corporation is a distinct legal entity under California law. A new corporation is born when its Articles of Incorporation and By Laws are filed with the Secretary of State. A group home corporation is not a business owned and operated by individuals per se but by a "board of directors" of the corporation. A non-profit (public benefit) corporation is different from a for-profit corporation in a sense that a for-profit corporation has owners whose goal is to create a profitable return on their investments while a non-profit corporation is created for charitable reason, (i.e., to benefit the public at large and not for personal gain of certain individuals). *In group home non-profit corporations most of these types of organizations are established for their charitable purpose which is stated in the mission statement which could include providing shelter, care and guidance to abused and neglected children.*

In incorporating a non-profit organization, here are some important things to consider:

1. Prepare articles of incorporation and file them with the Secretary of State in the state where the business is located.

2. Prepare organization by-laws.

3. Conduct an initial meeting of the board of directors. Items covered in the Agenda usually include the adoption of the bylaws of the corporation, election of the officers and planning a budget.

4. Apply for federal tax exemption from the Internal Revenue Service.

5. Apply for state tax exemption from the Franchise Tax Board.

What is an Article of Incorporation?

An Article of Incorporation identifies the organization, its status, identity of individuals responsible for the organization, its location of business and its mission. Information contained in the articles of incorporation will provide the Department information concerning who is ultimately responsible for which/what functions in the facility. This information is especially necessary when there are unresolved issues that may require immediate attention within the facility. The Department need to know who the contact person is with regard to the operation of the facility and who is responsible for the business operation in general.

In the application for filing of articles of incorporation, it must indicate the individual who is primarily responsible for the business operations, the authorized representative to sign documents and if there is a board resolution to support the designee.

In general, a residential care business other than a group home must indicate whether it is a corporation, a partnership or a limited liability corporation, sole proprietorship. It should also state in a public document the name of a designated representative and a description of his/her roles and responsibilities.

The filing of this document signifies the birth of a corporation as soon as the form is filed and registered with the Secretary of State. The Articles of Incorporation must include:

1) The official name of the corporation.

2) A statement that the corporation is a nonprofit or for profit and,

3) The name and address of a person in California who will accept legal notices (California Corporations Code Section 5130). There may be more information that is required depending on the type of entity, which, if not included in the articles of incorporation, it must be included in the bylaws.

Officers of the Corporation:

Just like most corporations/organizations, a non-profit corporation must have at least three officers: a **President** (Chairman of the Board), a **Secretary**, and a Chief Financial Officer **(Treasurer)** (California Corporations Code Section 5213). Officers (president, vice president, secretary, and treasurer) are in charge of carrying out the day-to-day business of the corporation. Their powers, duties and responsibilities are set by the articles of incorporation, bylaws, or by resolution of the board of directors. Officers owe a fiduciary duty to the corporation and must act honestly and for the best interest of the corporation. One person may fill one or more of the officer positions. However, the person or persons who hold (s) the offices of Secretary and Treasurer cannot also be President at the same time.

What is the Board of Directors?

The board of directors ("board") is the governing body of the corporation. The board consist of persons named in the articles of incorporation or bylaws or elected by the creators of the corporation and later board members to act as members of the board.

Composition of the Board

While it is convenient to have employees or relatives on board, it is not always in the corporation's best interest because these individuals are likely "interested persons." There is a built-in conflict of interest if too many directors receive money from the corporation or if too many directors are related to employees of the corporation. In the case of a non-profit organization, no more than 49% of the board of directors may be "interested persons." "Interested persons" include any director who has received payment for services rendered within the past 12 months whether as an employee (full or part time), independent contractor, or otherwise. If a director is related to anyone who has received payment from the corporation, that director may be an "interested person" (California Corporations Code Section 5227). There is a good reason for this rule. Directors may have to decide whether to use corporate money for their own personal purpose (or other interests) or for the corporation's charitable purposes. By limiting the number of "interested persons" serving as directors, the corporation limits the potential for self-dealing transactions and other conflict of interest.

Board of Directors Duties:

a. Select, employ, assess and, if necessary, dismiss the Chief Executive officer.

b. Provide support, comments and criticism, when needed; hold the staff accountable for carrying out plans and policy decisions; provide a formal performance review and appraisal.

c. Adopt and monitor the corporation's operating budget, financial development plan and insurance program.

d. Review and understand the financial statements on a regular basis to ensure the financial health of the corporation and that the corporate funds are managed appropriately and in accordance with the board's financial plan and budget.

e   Perform its legal responsibilities.

f   To act for the corporation as outlined in the articles of incorporation, constitution and/or bylaws.

g. Protect the assets of the corporation. Ensure that no board member, management, or staff is overpaid or unfairly or unreasonably profiting from business dealings with the corporation.

h. Ensure the corporation's equipment is not being misused. Ensure all purchases and leases have fair and reasonable terms, and represent the best deal possible to the corporation.

i. Board development (recruiting, orienting and assessing the board).

j   Aside from attending board meetings, it is also recommended that directors take the time to get to know about the group home facility and its needs. Conduct regular on-site facility visits. When appropriate, take the time to talk with the children and staff. This hands-on approach will provide valuable information about the operations of the group home.

k. Standard of Care. Directors must perform their duties in the following manner:

The duties must be observed in a manner that the director believes to be making decisions for the best interest of the corporation; and the duties must be performed with such care, including reasonable inquiry, required under the circumstances (California Corporations Code Section 5231).

The directors have the authority and responsibility for managing the non-profit corporation. The directors meet and make decisions together as the board of directors ("board"). The board is ultimately responsible for making sure a corporation is managed accordingly. If it fails to do so, individual directors may be held accountable. All corporate powers are exercised under the board's direction (California Corporations Code Section 5210). While certain powers may be assigned to committees, officers, or employees, their use of that power and their actions are subject to the board's review, direction and control. All day-to-day activities should be assigned to a particular staff member, or sometimes to the Executive Director, or to an administrator. While some important decisions may be delegated, those decisions must be reviewed and approved by the board. The board cannot simply give power and responsibility to the Executive Director and/or staff. The board and each director have a special legal relationship to the corporation. This relationship is known as "fiduciary relationship". As fiduciaries, directors must place the interests of the corporation before their own or others' interests. To protect the corporation's interest, the board must guard against harm to the corporation caused by any unfair or unreasonable transactions, conflict of interest or self-dealing transactions. To accomplish this, the board must take an active role in overseeing the corporation. The following are some specific duties of the board of directors:

- Prepare and approve long-range goals and objectives.

- Actively participate in the management, authorization of the corporation's long-term projection;

- Approve or delegate approval of annual objectives and priorities established to achieve long-range goals.

- Develop a financial plan to ensure that there are adequate funds to pay expenses and long-range goals and objectives. This could include fund raising to supplement the program.

- Make and adopt policies.

- Establish the limits of the Executive Director's authority to budget, administer finances and compensation, establish programs, and otherwise manage the corporation.

Minutes of the Board Meeting:

A non-profit corporation must keep a written record of the meetings of its board and committees of the board (California Corporations Code Section 6320). In addition, the minutes of the board meetings must be made available to California Department of Social Services staff upon request (Health and Safety Code Section 1520. l(f)). The law requires the minutes to contain enough information to make a clear written record for future use. The primary purpose for keeping minutes is to have documentation that explains the actions of the board, which later on can be used to defend their actions. Although minutes need not be a word-for-word record of everything said at a board meeting, they must present an accurate record of what was done, such as time, place, who was present, what was discussed, results of all votes taken, and what decisions were made and why. Also included are documentation procedures that the board or committee uses to make decisions (including financial statements) should be attached to the minutes if they are not confidential. If these documents are confidential, they must be clearly identified in the minutes. However, if the documents are usually a part of the corporation's permanent records, they must either be attached to the minutes or clearly identified in the minutes.

Usually the Secretary of the Corporation is responsible for preparing the minutes and distributes them either in advance of the next board meeting or at the meeting. A vote to approve the minutes is required only when board members want to make changes to the minutes as presented by the Secretary. Lastly, the minutes should be certified by the Secretary of the corporation (California Corporations Code Section 5215).

Board Meeting:

Board of directors meetings must be held at least every three (3) months (Health and Safety Code Section 1520.1 (e)). At these meetings, the board of directors shall review and discuss licensing reports (e.g. Compliant Report and Facility Evaluation Report), financial and program audit reports of its group home(s)/facility operations, incident reports filed with Community Care Licensing, and any administrative action against the licensee or its employees. It is acceptable to designate a board committee to review these documents and provide a full report to the board of directors. However, any discussions involving specific children/residents living in the group home/facility or specific employees must be kept confidential. Their names should not appear in the minutes. The minutes shall reflect the board's discussion of these documents and the facility/group home's operation.

Board of directors meetings can be held **anywhere** stated in the notice (including out of state or another country or even in a local restaurant or park), bylaws or board resolution. If the meeting place is not stated in any of these ways, then it must be held at the principal office of the corporation.

Voting Requirements:

In order for any act or decision of the board of directors to be official, it must be voted on by a quorum. A quorum is the number of members necessary to take action at a meeting (California Corporations Code Section 5211). The quorum may be stated in the articles of incorporation or bylaws and must meet the legal rules. A quorum can never be less than the majority of directors present.

Due Diligence:

In exercising due diligence, the directors must conduct a reasonable investigation into the facts. For example, assume the corporation is considering hiring one of its directors to perform bookkeeping services. An independent person or committee should be appointed to conduct an investigation into the facts. At a minimum, the facts considered should include what bookkeeping services are required and what other bookkeepers charge for similar services. The fair market rates should then be compared to that of the "interested director." The directors must review in good faith all the information gathered by the independent investigation, and all other relevant information, and ask all necessary questions in order to make an honest and informed decision. This review and comparison will indicate to the board whether the transaction is "fair and reasonable" to the corporation.

As a practical matter, thorough and complete board minutes should be kept of any board meeting where a self-dealing transaction is reviewed and approved. All information gathered by the independent review and any written reports relied upon by the directors should be included or attached to the minutes. The actions of the board must appear proper; the intent must be proper; and the outcome must be in the best interest of the corporation. If these actions are not performed, the transaction could project the appearance of fraud and collusion by the directors, and all directors could be held liable for damages to the corporation.

Improper transaction:

A loan made by a corporation to a director, officer, or relative of either, or a third party associated with those persons, may be improper. Directors may be held personally liable for making a loan of charitable assets. Prior approval from a court or the Attorney General is required for most loans from a public benefit corporation to an officer or director (California Corporations Code Section 5236).

Certain distribution of corporate assets is prohibited, such as: (1). transfers of corporate funds or assets to directors, officers, or members without fair consideration; (2). payment of excessive or unauthorized salaries or "bonuses";

Can a board ever approve a self-dealing transaction?

Not all self-dealing transactions are necessarily bad or unfair to the corporation. There may be cases where the self-dealing transaction benefits the corporation. For example, if a director contracts to rent real estate or personal property or to provide services at a fair price, if the terms of the contract are fair and reasonable to the corporation, if the contract is for the corporation's benefit (not the director's benefit), and if the corporation could not obtain a better arrangement with reasonable effort under the circumstances, there is likely no damage to the corporation from the self-dealing transaction.

The board may approve or "validate" a self-dealing transaction if, before entering the transaction or any part of it, all of the following requirements are found to be true:

The corporation entered into the transaction for its sole benefit and not for the benefit of the interested director; the transaction was fair and reasonable to the corporation at the time the corporation entered into it;

Before approving the transaction, the board considered alternative arrangements and in good faith found, after reasonable investigation, that a more advantageous arrangement under the circumstances from disinterested parties could not be found; and the board approved the transaction with knowledge of the director's interest and by a majority vote of the directors then in office, excluding the vote of the interested director(s) (California CorporationCode Section 5233).

If the directors have all of the facts before them, and find all of the above to be true, they may "validate" a self-dealingtransaction. Before validating a self-dealing transaction, the directors must exercise due diligence in making sure the transaction is fair and reasonable to the corporation.

To perform duties in good faith, the director must honestly evaluate situations. Decisions and actions must be in the best interest of the corporation (benefit the children/residents), not the interest of any other person or entity. Directors are expected to attend board meetings as well as read and understand the material sent to them. If there is something they do to understand, then it's their responsibility to make a reasonable inquiry, ask questions about it and discuss these issues with the other directors. Directors must carefully and honestly review transactions involving the corporation and other parties. Directors must ensure transactions are fair and reasonable and in the corporation's best interest, not the best interest of someone else. This honest review, inquiry, and protection of the best interests of the corporation is particularly important when the board is asked to review transactions involving the corporation and other parties.

What are By-Laws?

The bylaws provide the rules for governing and operating the corporation (California Corporations Code Section 5151). If you have this information in your articles of incorporation, you do not need bylaws. However, if you make any changes to your Articles of Incorporation, you must file the changes with the Secretary of State. Bylaws must state the number of directors of the corporation, unless stated in the articles. Unless restricted by law or the articles of incorporation, the board of directors can set, adopt and amend bylaw provisions.

The following are typical provisions included in bylaws:

1. The time, place, and method used to call meetings of members, directors, and committees.

2. The duties, powers, method of election and qualification of directors.

3. The length of directors' terms.

4. The manner of appointment, duties, compensation, and the length of officers' terms.

5. The requirements of reports to members.

6. The rules for admitting and removing members.

7. The appointment and authority of committees.

8. The special requirements for the percentage of member and director votes needed to take certain actions.

9. The number of directors needed to make a quorum.

Note: A Sample By-Laws available in Exhibit One of this book.

Where to keep the Articles of Incorporations and Bylaws?

Current copies of the articles of incorporation and bylaws must be kept at your principal California office (California Corporations Code Section 5160). A copy of the bylaws and articles of incorporation should be kept up to date by filing copies of amendments as they are adopted by resolutions of the board of directors (California Corporations Code Sections 5215 and 5810-5820).

The directors are given the authority and responsibility for managing the corporation. The directors meet and make decisions together as the board of directors ("board"). The board is ultimately responsible for making sure a corporation is managed accordingly. If it fails to do this, individual directors may be responsible. All corporate powers are exercised under the board's direction (California Corporations Code Section 5210). While certain powers may be assigned to committees, officers, or employees, their use of that power and their actions are subject to the board's review, direction and control.

The final action is to register the business entity with the Secretary of State of the county where the business is located. To register the organization, forms are available through the local county agencies and the Office of the Secretary of State.

Registration cost may vary from State to State so the reader is advised to contact their local State office that handles the registration of business organizations.

The life of a corporation begins upon the filing of articles of incorporation with the Secretary of State's office. Prior to filing the articles of incorporation, the following issues should be considered:

Where should I form the corporation?

Whatever you prefer, you can incorporate in any of the 50 states. Delaware is a popular choice because of its history, experience, recognition and pro-business climate. In fact, over half of the companies listed on the New York Stock Exchange are incorporated in Delaware. Recently, Nevada has also gained popularity due to its pro-business environment and lack of a formal information-sharing agreement with the IRS. Neither Delaware nor Nevada has corporate income taxes, and business filings in these states can usually be performed more quickly than in other states. Many people also choose to incorporate in their home state. Doing so may save them money because corporations are required to register as a "foreign corporation" in each state where they do business, and there is often no need to pay another person to serve as the registered agent. For example, a Delaware corporation that has its main business office in Texas must register as a "foreign corporation" with the Texas Secretary of State.

However, if your home state has a high corporate income tax or high state fee, and your corporation will not "do business" in the home state, it may be wise to incorporate elsewhere. "Doing business" means more than just selling products or making passive investments in that state. It usually requires occupying an office or otherwise having an active business presence.

Choosing a name

In general, the name of a corporation must end with "incorporated," "corporation," "corp." or "Inc." A name will not be accepted if it is likely to mislead the public or if it too closely resembles the name of another corporation formed in that state. If the name of your corporation will be used in connection with goods or services, you may wish to consider obtaining federal trademark protection for the name. This ensures that no one else in the U.S. may use that name in connection with the same general type of goods or services (except in areas where someone else is already using that name). Likewise, in establishing a residential care business, the name of the company may be different from the name of the facility. There is no requirement as to what names are allowed or not allowed. Most of the facilities I know are named after the streets where they are located, Saints or unusual names that are purely dependent on whatever a business owner can think of.

The Board of Directors

A corporation is managed by the board of directors, which must approve major business decisions. A director can be, but is not required to be, either a shareholder or an officer. Like representatives in congress, directors are elected by the shareholders and typically serve for a limited term. Each corporation must have at least one director.

Examples of procedures which must be approved by the board of directors include:

- Declaring a dividend
- Electing officers and setting the terms of their employment.
- Amending bylaws or the articles of incorporation .
- Any corporate merger, reorganization or other significant corporate transaction

Directors of a corporation owe duties of loyalty and care to the corporation. Generally, means that directors must act in good faith, with reasonable care, and in the best interest of the corporation.

Registered Agent

Each corporation must have a registered agent, the person designated to receive official state correspondence and notice if the corporation is "served" with a lawsuit. The registered agent must be either (1). An adult living in the state of formation with a street address (P.O. boxes are not acceptable) or (2). A corporation with a business office in the state of formation which provides registered agent services.

As previously mentioned, one of the advantages of forming a corporation in your home state is that any officer or director can act as the registered agent. However, there are some advantages to having another person or company act as your registered agent. First, this adds an extra layer of privacy, since the name and address of the registered agent is publicly available. Second, this ensures that if your corporation is named in a lawsuit, no one will surprise you at home on a Sunday night with court papers.

Corporations compared to LLCs

Limited liability companies are a relatively new type of business entity that combines the personal liability protection of a corporation with the tax benefits and simplicity of a partnership. However, there are still other important differences. The following discusses the main advantages and disadvantages of corporations versus LLCs.

Advantages of Corporations:

Profits are not subject to social security and medi-care taxes.
Salaries and profits of an LLC are subject to self-employment taxes. With a corporation, only salaries, and not profits, are subject to such taxes. This advantage is most significant for stockholder-owners who take a salary of less than $72,600.

For example, if an owner-employee of an LLC earns $40,000 in salary and is distributed $20,000 of the LLC's profits, a percentage tax would have to be paid on $60,000. For an S-corporation, social security and Medi-care taxes would only have to be paid on the $40,000 salary. This saves the stockholder-employee over $3,000 per year. Please note, however, that the IRS frowns upon employee-owners of an S-corporation not paying themselves salary and simply distributing the profits. In situations where the IRS feels that shareholders are taking too little in salary, the IRS will characterize all or part of the profits as salary.

Since limited liability companies are still relatively new, not everyone is familiar with them. In some cases, banks or vendors may be reluctant to extend credit to limited liability companies. Moreover, there are restrictions as to the type of business that an LLC may conduct in some states

Greater variety of, and fewer taxes on, fringe benefits. Corporations offer a greater variety of fringe benefit plans than any other type of business entity. Various retirements, stock option and employee stock purchase plans are available only for corporations. Plus, while sole proprietors, partners and employees owning more than 2% of an S-corporation must pay taxes on fringe benefits (such as group-term life insurance, medical reimbursement plans, medical insurance premiums and parking), stockholder-employees of a C-corporation do not have to pay taxes on these benefits.

Tax Flexibility: Although C-corporations are subject to double taxation, they also offer greater tax flexibility. A C-corporation does not have to immediately distribute its profits to shareholders as a dividend.

Disadvantages of Corporations

More corporate formalities: Corporations must hold regular meetings of the board of directors and shareholders and keep written corporate minutes. Members and managers of an LLC need not hold regular meetings, which reduce complications and paperwork.

Ownership restrictions for S-corporations: S-corporations cannot have more than 75 stockholders, and each stockholder must be an individual who is a resident or citizen of the United States. It is also difficult to place shares of an S-corporation into a living trust. None of these restrictions or difficulties applies to an LLC.

Shareholders of C-corporations cannot deduct operating losses. Members who are active participants in the business of an LLC are able to deduct operating losses of the LLC against their regular income to the extent permitted by law. Shareholders of an S-corporation are also able to deduct operating losses, but not shareholders of a C-corporation.

FICTITIOUS BUSINESS NAME

File for Fictitious Business Name Statement

After a company is registered with the Secretary of State, the next step is to apply for a fictitious business name statement to properly identify the applicant's business name. Technically, one may need to search whether the business name already exist and if it is, such name can not be used by another entity. In order to do this, the applicant must submit with the County Register's Office an application for a fictitious name business statement. The application will be published in a local newspaper to announce to the community that you are claiming a right over your business name. If no one comes forward to contest it within at least a couple of weeks or so, (typically 15 to 30 days) then the business name is officially registered under the same requested name. The application for filing a fictitious business name is normally held at the County Records Office in the local City Hall of the city in the county where the business will be established and there is a corresponding fee for the registration with the County Hall of Records. After registering your business name, you will be instructed to contact your local publication of your choice (for a fee) to publish your fictitious business name statement in the local newspaper to announce to the community of a newly established entity.

BUSINESS LICENSE

The next thing to do is to apply for a Business License in the city where you will conduct your business. For a set fee based on projected or actual income, a set fee schedule is available as a basis for the cost of your business license fee. Contact your local City Hall of Records for more information.

Secure your Tax Identification Number (TIN) and Employer's Identification Number (EIN) with the IRS and the Franchise Tax Board

After registering the business entity and filing for a fictitious business name statement, the next step shall be to contact your local Internal Revenue Service (IRS) to notify them about your new business. There is an automated number that you can contact or check your local phone directory listing for Government Agencies and look specifically for IRS. For convenience, one can register either by phone or online and you can secure your Tax Identification Number and Employers' Identification Number within minutes. Within 15 to 30 days, you will receive a confirmation letter indicating your official business numbers. These numbers are practically essential especially when you apply for tax exemption or tax benefits and also when you open a corporate account at a local banking institution and when you apply for a business license in the area where you want to establish the business.

OPEN A BUSINESS BANKING ACCOUNT

In order to fully function as a business, you need to have business banking capability to handle your financials, the deposits and the advances made through your venture capitalist and investors. You also might need an account to show your credit worthy enterprise. This is optional at this time as it is up to you to exercise the option as you will need to do it in the near future anyway, might as well do it now. In order to open an account with your local bank, you will need the following:

1. Articles of Incorporation and By-Laws registered with the Secretary of State.
2. Tax Identification Number/ Employer's Identification Number
3. Business License
4. A Board Resolution authorizing the opening of a business banking account.
5. Fictitious Business Name Statement
6. Business address
7. Other forms depending on the bank or institution.

Chapter 9: ACQUIRE THE PROPERTY/ BUSINESS

PURCHASING VS. LEASING THE PROPERTY /BUSINESS

One most important step that a start up residential care business would have to go through is the decision to buy or lease a property before submitting the application. In order to submit an application for a license to operate a facility, one of the requirements in the application is the address of the facility and proof of physical control of the property in a form of a title or a lease agreement. In order for an application to be processed, there must be a physical address of the "would be" facility. Even if the application for a license was submitted but without a property location, chances are the application will be returned to the sender or the process will be on hold until a location is specified in the application. There must be a facility location indicated in the application regardless whether the property is purchased or leased; in progress of being purchased or on lease. So, how can one submit an application for a license when the determination of property location is still in progress? Well, this is indeed a very difficult question to answer but it all depends on the situation. For instance, if an individual owns a certain residential property preferably a three bedroom home with at least one bath, even if it is a personal home, the applicant may be able to use it as the facility address and convert the home to meet the guidelines for residential care setting, then submit the application for processing. Even if the applicant is intending to purchase an already existing facility, the same principle applies. The applicant must be candid and honest by informing the licensing program analyst conducting the review that the current facility address is the temporary residence which will be converted into a facility or that the applicant is intending to purchase an already existing facility and the transition process is taking place.

However, if the applicant (like in most cases) do not have the house/ facility or physical address for the location of the facility, chances are that Community Care Licensing Program Analyst LPA reviewing the program design will not review the application and will place the application on hold or possibly deny the application until an address is finally determined. The reason in most cases is that LPA shall request for a fire marshal to visit and certify the location if it meets the standards for a residential care facility and that the LPA and the vendorizing agencies will need to send their representative to the location in order to determine if a temporary license is to be issued after meeting the guidelines.

What type of house is allowed in residential care setting, residential or commercial?

In most cases where small family homes, foster family homes and transition homes are concerned, the type of homes normally used are apartment units, condominium units, duplexes, triplexes and multi-family unit homes where the business can be started in a mixed use property like commercial/residential classification. However, in Group Homes, Residential Care Facilities for Adults and the Elderly, it is important that the facility structure must be (if possible) single story, single family home, detached multi-family unit homes, triplex and duplex homes for practical reasons such as cost effective management, ease in supervision and monitoring of clients safety, accessibility and mobility as primary reasons.

What and where is a good location to put up a residential care facility?

Just like any business, location is extremely important. Before making any major property purchase/lease, the applicant must first get in contact with placing agencies and licensing agencies and find out what and where is a good location. They have a better idea on what part of the county is already saturated with the same services that you might be offering, so in order to avoid overcrowding in one certain area, it is wise to seek assistance. Another important factor that could affect the location of your business is the guarantee of continued referrals from placement agencies. Almost all agency referrals are very dependent on factors such as location and type of facility, quality and the variety of the service, consistency in the delivery of the quality service to the clients/consumers etc... The key is that the facility must be established in an area where there is high demand for the type of service.

The choice of facility location is also dependent on how accessible it is to the community resources such as fire department, schools,

YMCA, market, police, jobs, groceries, hospitals and clinics etc... that will be accessible to the consumers living in the facility.

Step 6: Acquire the Business/Real Estate property on lease or purchase

Q: If there is someone selling a residential care business in the area, is it a good idea to buy the business instead of starting from scratch?

A: Buying an existing facility has its advantages and disadvantages just like everything else. One of the fastest and the shortest way to start this business is of course buying an already existing facility with available clients being served. As you know, the whole initial process could take another six (6) months to one (1) year to market the business before you will be able to attain positive cash flow in your business unless there is an emergency placement. Meanwhile, you will be saving a lot of time and effort when you just take over the management and ownership of an already existing business/facility. All you need to do is to continue on with what was left for you to do by the previous owner. Purchasing an already existing business is the most common way of starting this business the easy way. If you are lucky to buy a well kept business and has already existing clients, it is good, but quite challenging in a long term because if you do not know the history of the facility or the company that you are dealing with, then you are up to a lot of surprises.

Remember that when you buy an already existing business, it must prove its potentials first and that there are clients being served already, that all you need to do is to continue the service. When you buy the business, you only buy the real estate property and the potentials for income of the business. Do not presume that with the sale of the business comes with it the sale of the clients. The sale of the business does not always come with a guarantee that the residents remain where they are. They have the option to move or be transferred by their respective social workers or relatives if they choose to do so. That is why you have to be honest and be careful when you buy an already existing business. By informing the representatives as well as the licensing offices in advance to make them aware of your pending sale transaction, there will be no surprises. If you are not honest with your transaction, you might be the one who is in for the big surprise. But as a word of caution, if you are planning to do it this way, remember the following:

1. Check the financial feasibility of the business.
2. Verify the credibility of the selling company/individual
3. Review its history, past incidences, current relationship with the licensing / placement agencies with the past operator.
4. Analyze the experiences, education, training and qualification of the former owner.
5. Review records, evaluate business management skills and current community relations of the selling company.
6. Is the license current and does the company owe fees and costs from past deficiencies.
7. Evaluate past debts and review viability
8. Etc..

Have you tried buying a used car or house in your life?

The experience is similar to that parallel where the buyer does not know what happened in the past, what is the real reason why the business is being sold and for what purpose. As you know, buying an exiting business is great but be very careful.

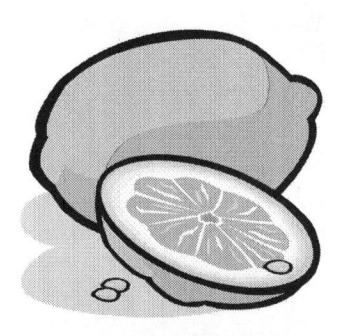

Remember to do the following first before you sign the contract of sale:

- Consult with your Licensing Program Analyst LPA.

- Be honest and candid by telling your LPA in advance that you are planning to buy or sell an existing facility. They will work with you on this by giving you advice and consultation on what you need to do.

- Check the website of California Association of Health Facilities CAHF at http://www.cahf.org/ to verify current standing of the facility that you are interested in.

- Pre-qualify the seller. It also means that you as the buyer will need meet the minimum requirement in setting up the facility. You will need to prove your experience, your specialized training and possibly undergo orientation just like everybody else.

- Check title on the property, go to the city hall and research with the county register of deeds, tax department, check for liens, attachments, unpaid bills, questionable ownership of title, etc...

- Do your homework and protect your rights.

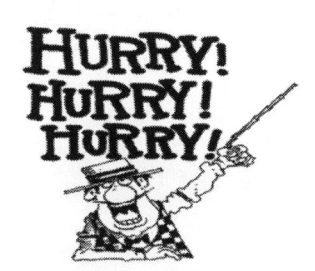

HURRY! HURRY! HURRY!

Advertisement:

Wanted: BUYER FOR A 6 BED. LEVEL 2 RESIDENTIAL CARE FACILITY FOR THE DEVELOPMENTALLY DISABLED ADULTS. ANNUAL INCOME POTENTIAL UP TO $400K. CONTACT OWNER. (800)123-4567. Desperately seeking interested buyers

Once in a while, you will come across in newspapers or magazine advertisements similar to what is shown in this page or you meet a friend who knows someone in the business selling their business. Well, to those who have cash and are ready to go, this is not a bad idea if you are too eager to get things going. But, you have to remember and ask yourself these questions:

1. Why is it for sale and for what price?
2. How long has it been in the market and how long have they been in business?
3. Is there a problem or are there potential problems apparent in the operations of the business?
4. What are possible factors behind the selling of the business?

5. What is current relationship of the owner with the licensing and other placement agencies?
6. What is its annual income as compared to its annual expenses?
7. Where is the area and how is the condition of the property?
8. Is it worth it?
9. Does the facility qualify to meet the buyer's expectations of a successful business.

Buying an already existing business may not be a bad idea for those who are in a hurry and want to jump into the next available business opportunity right away. Caution: Be very careful. Caveat Emptor "Buyers Beware". You need to know what exactly you are getting into, if you don't, you have to hold on and get things straight before you draw that check to pay off the transaction. The sample questions raised earlier are important points to think about but not necessarily the only things to consider as your individual cases may vary. Always remember to contact your local licensing office and do your research on the facility that you are considering.

- Take a look at the facility's background, history, incident reports, complaints, violations, deficiencies;
- Interview the staff, talk to the residents, interact with the neighbors,
- Get some references, check with health care licensing, community care licensing,
- Check with the local police and other enforcement agencies, talk to the fire marshal and learn more about the physical plant of the facility,
- Review their financial statement, dig through the records,
- Observe signs that might give you some doubts, abuse reports, deficiency reports, reported and unreported incidences such as death, injuries, accidents, etc...
- Check the license if it is still valid, and lots of questions to answer before you draw that check.
- Do everything you need to do to satisfy your interest and ask the help of a consultant in the business.

As a buyer you must also have a purchase agreement which must specify a window period when you may have the option to back out of the transaction should the facility is unable to meet the regulation guideline or that the sale must be subject to certain conditions such as approval of a business loan, approval of the sale of the business by the licensing agency as well as the placement agency, subject to the buyer being approved or qualified by licensing agency etc.. "before the actual transaction is considered final". For your peace of mind,you the buyer must come up with contingency provisions to be able to back out from a deal that is relatively fraudulent. Be careful of fraudulent or seemingly fraudulent transactions because eventually, the truth will come out and you as the unsuspecting applicant/buyer will bear all the burden of moving on with the problems of the facility when the transaction becomes final.

There are some facilities being offered for sale due to retirement or illness of its operator/licensee, lack of funding, death in the family etc.. Each situation may vary as there is no right or wrong answer to this question. It is purely up to the buyer of the business to make that determination. The buyer alone can answer their own honest question. "When in doubt, check it out".

On the subject of **LOCATION** for the facility, it is a good idea to first check with your local placement agency, community care licensing office, city council of the area where the facility might be located; consider proposed state and federal mandates and regulations affecting the use of properties in certain areas before going beyond application stage. There may be some restrictions on the conditional use of the properties in certain areas and there may be a limit as to the number of facilities allowed at a given time, location and purpose.

Depending on concurrent state and federal funding and budget allocations, setting up of a new facility in a local area may definitely have an impact on the future facility operators. That is why, my suggestion is to initially contact the agencies whom the applicant is planning to deal with such as Regional Centers, Dept. of Mental Health, Dept. of Aging, Probation etc.. to find out where is a good area of preference and what type of facilities that are available for funding. Once a suggested location is determined, then there is some form of an assurance that the applicant is on the right track. Research for the right location before you make the purchase or sign up that lease agreement. Find out the market for the business, talk to your competition if any, make your plans.

The 300 Feet Rule:

In order to prevent over population and saturation of identical services in one concentrated single area, Community Care Licensing came up with the "300 feet Regulation" whereby any new facility in a given area may not be located within no less than 300 feet from the next facility of the same or identical service facility unless it is owned and operated by one and the same owner or organization.

The reason behind this is that most city councils, planning commission and licensing agencies does not allow over crowding in certain residential and commercial areas to avoid congestion or traffic, to control the mushrooming of facilities which could affect the community in particularly safety, availability of resources, education and human services, domestic management and control and possible neighborhood complaints. There is nothing wrong for a company or an individual to establish five different facilities in one square block as long as there is neighborhood and city council approval. There has been horrible stories where a home was forced to shut down due to pressure from neighbors and the city council. Make sure you have all the proper clearances and check things out with your neighbors and find out what they feel about your plan to set up a facility that could have an impact in their community.

LEASE WITH OPTION TO PURCHASE:

Have you considered leasing a property for use as a facility?

The idea of leasing a property specially at the beginning stage of the business may be a very good idea particularly if you have limited capital, as long as you inform the landlord/owner outright about the intent of the lease. Depending on what the seller's situation is, most of the time, sellers will be willing to become a landlord initially and then eventually become the seller. Most of the times, the seller is willing to work things out to benefit both the buyer and the landlord/seller. Depending on every situation, it is always wise to consult an

Attorney or a professional when it comes to your individual situation. Each situation is unique and it deserves a unique preparation plan.

For those who do not have enough capital to start the business, have you considered leasing the property initially and perhaps later on exercise your option to purchase the property when the business is starting to generate revenues? This practice is commonly called **"LEASE WITH OPTION TO PURCHASE"** which to some people makes a lot of sense because it has considerable advantages but with only quite a few disadvantages.

Advantages of Leasing a Property:

1. Low initial capital requirement.
2. Limited commitment which means that when you decide that the business is not working out right and you suddenly want to give it up or sell the business, you will only lose a very minimal amount which is practically your earnest money deposits.
3. Sometimes if you can work out a deal whereby the owner can include the furniture and appliances as part of the lease.
4. You will have the option to own a property with little or no money down depending on your deal with the property owner.

Disadvantages:

1. Practically, none. If you are unable to meet the contract requirement to exercise your option, you might lose the lease deposits, earnest money or you can ask for extensions if possible.
2. You have to qualify based on your credit history and capacity to meet your obligation.

If you do not have a lot of money to start with, leasing may be a good alternative. On your lease-purchase agreement, you must specify in a statement that says "with option to purchase" to be transparent in the transaction. A key ingredient is for you the future owner of the property to make sure that you like the property first. You must have a long term plan to recoup your investment by considering property values or future potential of the area location. The property must have a good property valuation reflected on the appraisal report. Most importantly, you must find the right landowner who will work things out with your plan. On this subject, I suggest that you look for a good realtor and a knowledgeable real estate attorney who can negotiate and draw a good contract just for your purpose. Personally, to me leasing at the beginning is a better way to go than buying a property especially for those who do not have enough money to work with. All you need is a deposit and negotiate the right monthly payment that will blend well with your projected revenues. Remember what was said about preparing a business plan, at this point, the plan can be very useful.

On the other hand, for those of you who already have the real estate property intended for this purpose, it will be easier because practically, you are just expanding the revenue potential of the property that you have by making use of it and generating annual deductibles in return. Talk to your financial adviser and find out more on this. Most of the people I know who started in the business prefer leasing, then after a couple of years when the business takes off, they exercise their option of purchasing the property.

Things to consider when buying a property for the business

1. Location must be accessible to transportation, parks and recreation, library, school, police, market activities etc..
2. Look for a house that is low in maintenance and repair.
3. Consider a home that has potential for high resale value
4. There is no rule on whether a home/facility should have a second floor but depending on the type of consumers to supervise and their restricted health conditions or behavior, a one-floor home may be an excellent choice for obvious reasons and one of them is staff/owner operator accessibility to the consumer to be effectively supervised and monitor their needs.
5. Homes must be well kept and clean at all times.
6. The home must be fire proof-ready with sprinklers and alarms.

7. The size of the home must be generous to moderate and its smallest room must preferably be no smaller than 10 Feet X 12 feet in size.
8. The home must preferably be in a good area or neighborhood.

SALE-LEASE BACK

Sale-lease back is a term used when a property is sold by the SELLER to a BUYER and then turns back around to take possession of the property as a TENANT of the same property for a given fee or consideration. The SELLER wants to retain possession of the property by leasing it back from the BUYER for a considerable amount as a lease payment, make exclusive use of the property and in the short term future (perhaps after three years or more), SELLER would like to exercise the option of buying back the property at an agreed amount or price. This is another creative form of financing where a property owner makes use of its available equity by pulling out cash from the sale proceeds of the property, using the same cash for the business operations, declares the lease as an expense and get the benefit of tax deductibles of leasing as a business. Then at the end of the lease when the business takes off, buys back the property. This approach may not be applicable to everyone so, please consult with a real estate attorney who may have other ideas applicable to your particular financial situation. There are other creative ways you can fund your business. You either use equity on a property or use other people's funds if you know what I mean. There are also self-help books available at the bookstore and the internet on financing a business.

Chapter 10: THE HOST LETTER

Step 7: Secure Host Letter

Securing a host letter shall be optional in some cases depending on the type of facility being set up as well as the county where the business will be located. It is highly recommended however that an applicant should always secure host letter from the city or county of business to inform them as well as the community that there will be a new business in the area that could affect the neighborhood in general.

As a start up facility, it is always a good practice to introduce yourself to the community and notify your future neighbors about your plan to establish a business of caring for individuals in a residential care setting. Before you physically locate your business, especially for day care centers and day programs including care homes where the community may be affected, it is courtesy to acknowledge the people around you who could have some impact in your business as well as the impact of your business to the community.

Most of the times, there are no objections but there are quite a few isolated situations when the city council may refuse to issue a permit to operate a day care center in areas sensitive to public safety and the community interest. Whenever you encounter some form of opposition from the community, you will normally be invited to attend a community meeting that is held typically in a town hall in the presence of the community representatives, city council members, the mayor and all other entities that could be affected by your future business. It is a matter of reaching out to the community and address their issues and opinion and to explain how they will benefit from your facility.

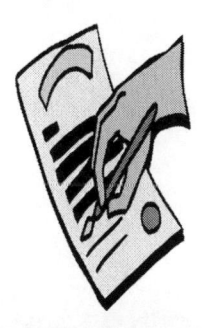

Chapter 11: INSURANCE COVERAGE

Step 8: Get your facility insured

Living in a "lawsuit-happy" society, we all have to be very cautious particularly with the way we do business of caring for others. All businesses regardless of its nature and scope must have an insurance coverage to protect itself from fraudulent and opportunistic transactions. If you are already in business and do not have any form of insurance coverage to back you up, you might have a problem. Let us take for example the situations of residential care facilities where people and families are involved, insurance coverage is "a must" to cover for future incidences or else expect a total wipe out of your business long before you even start breaking even.

An important element in avoiding lawsuit is your efficient management and administration. Along with it is the sufficient training of your staff, proper monitoring and documentation and of course the continuing education. Despite of meticulous risk management and prevention, accidents do happen therefore, insurance coverage will come in handy in times when you needed it.

First, let us start with your biggest investment your property. You need to cover it with property insurance for accidental falls, theft, fire, death and calamity.

Secondly, you need to cover your business and yourself from fraudulent and malicious claims from clients or staff by acquiring professional and general liability insurance to cover liabilities at a minimum of $1 Million Dollars in claims for abuse and allegations, etc..

Thirdly, you need to cover your staff with claims and workers compensation, disabilities insurance etc…

Fourthly, if you will be transporting clients on a regular basis, you will need to have comprehensive transportation coverage and third party liability insurance.

And, last but not the least secure other blanket insurance to cover you and your business as well as future earnings. If you do not, you are leaving your operations to chance and chances are you can't fight chance with a hope and a prayer. Secure your business first. Besides, the vendoring agencies will require a proof of current coverage before they will send you their referrals/business.

THE APPLICATION PACKET
Chapter 12: SUBMITTING THE APPLICATION PACKET

Step 9: Submit the Application for a License to Operate a Facility. (Second Stage/Component)

The next step is for you to apply for a license to operate the facility by going to the Community Care Licensing office CCL and to get an application packet. You can also secure the forms through the Internet website of CCL by entering the California Department of Social Services and gain access to the state website.

Included in the application packet are the following set of information that you might need to enclose as part of your documentations before submitting the application back to Licensing:

1. Application Form
2. Application Processing Fee (Depending on facility type, estimated number of occupants/bed etc..)
3. Proof of Entity / Corporation (Non-profit / For Profit)
4. Franchise Tax / IRS
5. Employment Identification Number
6. Administrator Certificate
7. Business license
8. Bank account and statement of deposit
9. Certification of available funds from the bank
10. Health certificate, TB-HIV Test
11. Live-Scan Fingerprint Clearances
12. Facility location
13. Facility sketch of the internal and external description
14. Emergency Plan
15. Disaster Plan
16. Emergency Intervention Plan
17. Business Forms
18. Operations manual
19. Business location
20. Fire Marshall Certificate (if available)
21. Host Letter (if available)

22. Bond
23. General, Professional Liability Insurance and other related coverage
24. Transportation plan
25. Program Design
26. Staff Schedule
27. Sample menu
28. Interim Activity Schedule

While the application is under review with the Community Care Licensing, it is very important for you the applicant to know that the process could take at least 90 days from the date of submission before a response or approval, denial or revision of documentation could take place. It is also important for you to respond within 30 days from the date of receipt of correction or denial otherwise, the application may be rejected for lack of interest.

To some of you who are responding to a Request for a Proposal RFP, let me remind you that the initial process all the way up to submission of program design may be different depending on individual situation. In the next chapter, there will be a brief discussion on the difference between going through the normal application process and comparing it with the process undertaken when responding to a Request for Proposal RFP.

FIRE MARSHAL CERTIFICATION

Step 10: Request for Fire Marshal to Inspect the Facility and Request for Certification

Upon acquisition of a facility location whether it be intended for residential care facility or commercial use such as a day care center for seniors or adults, the next plan of action is to have the location certified appropriately for the intended purpose. For most recently built homes or facilities, chances are they are equipped with fire sprinklers, exits, alarms and smoke detectors. However, for those that were built without it are required to meet the minimum guideline for safety especially for the disabled and the seniors depending on the county or city where the facility is located. Consult with your local fire department and the community care licensing as far as the requirements are for the general area where your facility will be located. Retrofitting a home to meet the guideline can be costly at times so, make sure that you have the right stuff in the home before you make your purchase. It is also a good idea to hire the services of a professional property inspector to evaluate the property to meet the standards for safety regulation.

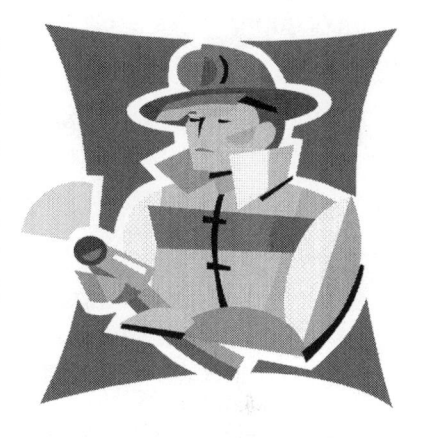

As soon as you have the property location for your business, request for a fire marshal inspection which may be arranged through the assistance of Community Care Licensing who sets up the appointment to visit your facility. The inspector will provide the certification if it meets the minimum standard allowable as far as the number of occupants in the house and the type of population, ambulatory or non-ambulatory etc... that will be using the facility.

Depending on various factors, the inspection could take at least 15 to 30 days on schedule for the fire marshal to physically inspect the property and perhaps wait for another 15 days before a certification letter may be issued in your favor as the applicant, indicating whether the property is appropriate as a facility or not. During the inspection, the fire marshal may review the in-house copy of the structural plan and design, the electrical and structural components, and physically inspect and evaluate the property for physical site problems that could pose as a danger to the safety and well- being of its occupants. As soon as the certificate is ready, a copy shall be mailed to the applicant as well as the licensing agency.

Important things to remember:

1. Each bedroom no matter what size and structure may not accommodate more than two occupants at any time.

2. Design the house/facility to accommodate mostly non-ambulatory consumers. In a non-ambulatory room, both ambulatory and non-ambulatory residents may use it, the room can be used as an alternative room for ill residents. That means more potential referrals can be accommodated in your facility.

3. Check the fire sprinkler system, extinguishers and exit accessibility. When looking for a prospective location to use as a facility, if possible, look for homes/structures that have already-installed fire sprinklers, smoke detectors and smoke alarms.

4. Prepare an Emergency Plan and Procedure which include an emergency temporary relocation site in case of fire, flood, natural calamities, etc... Emergency Intervention Plan for residents with special needs.

While waiting for fire marshal certification and application review, your next move at this point might be to advertise in the local newspaper for job applicants for possible hiring, advice your consultants to be ready to report for work upon license approval.

As the process could take a while (90 days or more) before everything is completed, advertising to hire temporary and on-call staff would be an excellent plan because when you reach this stage of the application process, it is almost close to its completion and that your facility must be ready to accommodate possible referrals from different agencies even

on short notices. Despite of the fact that your license is still pending review, one of the conditions for the success of your business is your ability to accommodate clients/referrals on an emergency basis should the need arise at a very short notice. It is always best to be prepared even if you have to pre-condition the facility as if it can accommodate the consumers even by tonight should there be a need.

REQUEST FOR PROPOSAL
Chapter 13: RESPONDING TO A REQUEST FOR PROPOSAL (RFP)

Q&A on Request for a Proposal

Q: What is a Request for a Proposal (RFP)?

A: Public agencies and other organizations from time to time solicit for Request for a Proposal RFPs with the public and its vendors to get quotes and bids on certain services or facilities that are unavailable at the time of request. Everyone who is expected to respond to the RFP must submit written suggestions, solutions, ideas and projects proposals on a specified format requirement to address issues that the agencies would like to resolve.

Q: How are bids evaluated?

A: Bids are usually evaluated based on several factors such as price, cost effectiveness of the proposal, experience and consistency of the respondents and their ability to meet the requirements and specifications of the RFP.

Bids for proposals are evaluated based on criteria specified by the soliciting agency and a composite score is developed with the lowest or highest evaluation being considered the best bid. There are a lot of different factors and ways to weight the evaluation. Interested parties, respondent/vendors usually want to know the criteria before they bid. It is important that the acceptance criteria must match the evaluation criteria to assure fair and high quality procurement. In responding to RFP's, the steps and preparation procedures may be different from those enumerated in this book, however the information discussed here is geared more towards describing a generalized procedure expected of most RFP's. *Do not confuse this procedure with the standardized preparation procedures in acquiring a licensed facility.*

There are only few exceptions that make RFP procedure different from the standard preparation in applying for a license.

Q: How is it different from the steps 1-10 we just discussed?

A: Responding to an RFP sometimes totally changes the process of establishing the residential care business. An individual or entity responding to RFP does not need to be licensed initially, does not initially need to have a program design available, does not need to have a facility location etc... before responding to an RFP. In short, anyone can respond with just an idea on paper and then work things out from the proposed idea. The first thing to do in responding to an RFP is to submit a proposal on how to resolve the issues stated in the request for a proposal. Only when the proposal has been deemed approved or acceptable will the responding individual or entity initiate the whole process mentioned in this book. With this in mind, there is the upside and the downside in an RFP. Advantages include the assurance of a guaranteed business from the proposing agency, possible start-up funding through grants to meet initial operating expenses in setting up the facility, the amount of risk is greatly reduced to an acceptable level and perhaps the whole undertaking is less tedious but the basic process remains the same. The disadvantages however, may include the fact that the individual is very much dependent on the grace and the mercy of the funding/approving agency, that even if the proposal is approved, there is still no guarantee that the business will continue to receive exclusive referral businesses from the approving agency, that if the individual does not meet the expectations specified in the contract of services (RFP), the facility is vulnerable to immediate shut down due to lack of consistent business referrals.

When a bid is accepted, the respondent shall submit a program design indicating how the ideas in the proposal shall be implemented, and if it requires a specific type of home, facility or equipment, the soliciting agency may at times provide start up funding for the purchase of the facility or services in a form of loan or grants.

Upon purchase or acquisition, the facility shall be licensed and while in progress, the operator and its staff may be provided with all the much needed service training on the operation of the facility/equipment in order to make the proposal complete.

Sometimes, RFP's do not provide start up funding but they guarantee consistent supply of business. The proposed provider shall submit all the required documentations similar or identical to the standardized requirements expected from those who normally apply for a license to operate a facility. The provider is required to under go identical processes such as orientations, training requirements, standard documentations, etc... The good part of it is that, since the approved provider becomes an acknowledged vendor for the requesting agency, in some ways or the other, the agency might be able to waive certain conditions that are normally required in order to facilitate the establishment or creation of the proposed facility/service with greater ease and flexibility. Upon procurement of all the necessary documentation specified in the requirements for licensing, a completed application may then be submitted for processing.

While awaiting licensing approval, the applicant may have the option to secure vendorization also known as accreditation to be able to receive consumer referrals from agencies such as Regional Centers, Probation, DCFS, CPS, APS etc...

If the individual or corporation will only accommodate private paying clients such as those who will live in facilities for the elderly, then vendorization may not be necessary.

What is vendorization and what does it take to become vendorized provider?

On the succeeding chapter, there will be a discussion on the subject of vendorization and its importance in the business.

Chapter 14: VENDORIZATION

Step 11. Secure Vendorization Packet:

In order to receive consistent referrals/clients from different placement agencies such as Regional Centers, Probation, Dept. of Aging, etc... a facility must be vendorized with the placing agency.

What is Vendorization ?

In order to meet the much needed services in the community, agencies provide vendorization. Vendorization is the process for identification, selection, and utilization of service providers based on the qualifications and other requirements necessary in order to maintain the standard and quality of services provided. The vendorization process allows placing agencies such as Dept. of Mental Health, Dept. of Aging, Dept of Social Services, Regional Centers to verify, prior to the provision of services to consumers, that an applicant for vendorization meets all of the requirements and standard specified in the regulations. Applicants who meet the specified requirements and standards are assigned a service code and a unique vendor identification number in order to receive business from designated public agencies.

Service providers are vendored by the soliciting agency whose allocated catchment area covers the location where the service is originating from. Placement referrals in residential care facilities may come not only from the vendoring catchment region/areas but also from other sources or regions in need of a particular service.

Does the facility have to be licensed first before being vendorized or approved facility?

YES. One of the major requirements of placement agencies is that, in order to be vendorized and to start receiving referrals, the facility must first have a valid license. The exception to the general rule is expected in cases of RFP's which was discussed earlier. In most cases, other agencies such as Regional Centers, Dept. of Probation etc... are prohibited from referring any consumer to a facility until the vendor application is approved. However, if the placing agency determines that the health or safety of a consumer is in jeopardy, and no current vendor is available to provide the needed service, the Regional Center may have the option to approve emergency vendorization of a certain type of facilities in order to meet the needs of the clients.

Emergency vendorization allows placing agencies to approve vendorization of an applicant prior to completion of the vendorization process if the placing agency determines that the health or safety of a consumer is at risk and no current vendor is available to provide the much needed service. When the emergency vendorization is approved, the applicant may provide services for no more than 45 days, after which the emergency vendorization will lapse if the placing agency like Regional Center does not approve vendorization within 45 days of the initial authorization. If a lapse of emergency vendorization occurs, the vendor will not be allowed to reapply for emergency vendorization.

What is Regional Center?

Regional Center is a non-profit agency established in the State of California that promote and advocate for the rights of individuals with developmental disabilities defined under the Lanterman Act.

The State of California has a commitment to provide service and support to individuals with developmental disabilities throughout their lifetime. These service and support are provided through a combination of federal, state, county and local government services, private businesses, support groups and volunteers.

The Department of Developmental Services provides leadership and funding for these service and support through state-operated developmental centers and contracts with twenty-one agencies called Regional Centers.

The Regional Centers have offices throughout California to provide a local resource to help find, create and access the many services available to individuals with developmental disabilities and their families.

Regional Centers provide or coordinate the following services for individuals with developmental disabilities and their families:

> Information and referral
> Assessment and diagnosis
> Counseling
> Lifelong individualized planning and service coordination
> Purchase of necessary services included in the individual program plan
> Resource development
> Outreach
> Assistance in finding and using community and other resources
> Advocacy for the protection of legal, civil and service rights
> Early intervention services for at risk infants and their families
> Genetic counseling
> Family support
> Planning, placement, and monitoring for 24-hour out-of-home care
> Training and educational opportunities for individuals and families
> Community education about developmental disabilities

The vendoring Regional Center is responsible for ensuring that the applicant meets licensing, Title 22 and Title 17 requirements for vendorization, determining the appropriate vendor category for the service to be provided, and approving or disapproving vendorization based upon their review of the documentation submitted by the applicant.

Requirements of Becoming A Regional Center Vendorized Residential Care Service Provider

As mentioned earlier, there are advantages of being an accredited service provider for any public agency. One of these so-called public agencies is Regional Center. The following information is provided for those interested in operating a residential facility under the Regional Center catchment areas.

1. Prospective providers are expected to hold a minimum of six (6) months of prior direct care experience working with people with developmental disabilities in accordance with The California Code of Regulations, Title 17, Section 56037(b):

2. Attend orientation provided by Community Care Licensing (CCL). All communities in regional areas must call CCL or their local community care licensing office as well as their local Regional Center representatives to find out current schedules of specific business orientations. Example: A "small family home" serves children 0-17 years and the owner/licensee and his/her family may live on the premises. A "group home" also serves children 0-17 years but is normally run by staff. An "adult residential facility" serves individuals from 18-59 years of age. An "elderly facility" is for seniors who are 60 and above.

3. Attend and complete the "New Service Provider's Orientation" offered through your local Regional Center by contacting the resource development and training unit. There is a fee for the New Residential Service Provider Class. (Call your local agency for cost).

4. Obtain and read Title 17 Residential and Quality Assurance Regulations Section 56001-56207. A copy of Title 17 may be obtained at the DDS website (www.dds.ca.gov).

5. When selecting your facility, take into consideration that the real estate property you selected must at least be licensed for non-ambulatory residents because it is more likely to get referrals from Regional Center than facilities that can only accommodate for ambulatory residents. It is also suggested that you work with the Resource Development team to ensure that the proposed facility meets the currently identified service needs.

6. The applicant for vendorization must complete the CCL application process. Regional Center will only accept licenses which specify that the licensee prefers to serve developmentally disabled residents (Note: Residential care facilities for the

Elderly (RCFE) do not have a population identified on their license).

7. Submit proposed program design and a written request to your local Regional Center to establish an approved ARM (Alternative Residential Model) service level. The written request must include a statement of the administrator's qualifications.

8. Reference letters from three individuals or companies.

Reminder: Experience working with individuals with developmental disabilities is required BEFORE participation in the New Service Provider Orientation.

Experience requirement:

(a). Level 1-2: minimum 6 months experience.
(b). Level 3: minimum 9 months of experience
(c). Level 4: minimum 12 months of experience

9. Regional Center will review proposed Program Design within 45 days of receipt (in accordance with the California Code of Regulations, Title 17, Section 56005(3)(b)).

10. To successfully complete the New Vendor / Administrator interview.

11. Successfully complete an on-site facility review and complete the vendor application.

12. Successful completion of all the above requirements does not guarantee referral or placement of residents in the facility (Title 17, Section 54322). The maximum vendored capacity for all residential care facilities is four (4) beds per Welfare and Institutions Code, Section 4648(a)(3)(D) and Senate Bill 1038.

How does one become a Vendor?

To become a vendor of Regional Center, a Vendor Application (Form DS 1890) (form available through Regional Center) must be submitted along with the documentation specified in Title 17, Section

54310. Once a potential service provider has obtained all necessary licenses, submitted a complete application and all necessary documentation to the vendoring Regional Center, the Regional Center has 45 days to approve or disapprove vendorization. Once vendored, the service provider may be utilized by other Regional Centers, known as "user" or "utilizing" Regional Centers, as well as the vendoring Regional Center. The vendor identification number assigned by the vendoring Regional Center must be used by all Regional Centers purchasing the vendored service.

Although a Regional Center must vendor an applicant who meets all the requirements for the service to be provided, vendorization in no way obligates that Regional Center to purchase service from that vendor. For Children Adults/Senior Facilities, in order to be a vendorized provider/facility, the applicant must schedule with the respective agency responsible for placing consumers to the facility such as Dept. of Children and Family Services, Child Protective Services, Adult Protective Services, Dept. of Aging, Regional Center, Dept. of Mental Health etc.. to secure an appointment for an interview as to how one will present the benefits of using your facility or services.

Typically, appointment is set thru the placement agency who just like licensing offices, they will send a representative to inspect the facility. Should the facility as well as the program meets the standards of expectation set forth in the regulations, the agency shall conduct an orientation with the applicant to discuss their standards and expectations needed to benefit the consumers in the placement. In some agencies, orientation may take place for at least forty (40) hours depending on the type of facility and services offered. In order to be vendorized, the facility must offer the services that are expected and to maintain the standard of care based on the regulations. Most of the times, orientations are held at the local offices of the placing agencies. Upon satisfactory completion of the requirements set forth by the placing agencies, consumer placements shall take in effect as soon as possible. Most of the times, placement could take longer than one year depending on the given situation or circumstances.

The Vendorization Process :

An applicant who desires to be vendored shall submit Form DS 1890 (12/92), entitled Vendor Application, and the information specified in (1) through (10) below, as applicable, to the vendoring Regional Center.

1. Applicant's name including the governing body/organization
2. Applicant's Social Security/Federal Tax ID
3. Applicants Address
4. Address of Service
5. Name of owner or executive director;
6. Types of service to be provided;
7. Telephone number;
8. Facility capacity, if applicable;
9. Identification of the type of consultants, subcontractors and community resources to be used by the vendor as part of its service.
10. Copies of:

    (a). Any license, credential, registration, certificate or permit required for the performance or operation of the service, or proof of application for such document;

    (b). Any academic degree required for performance or operation of the service;

    (c). Any waiver from licensure, registration, certification, credential, or permit from the responsible controlling agency;

    (d). The proposed or existing program design as required in Sections 56712 and 56762 of these regulations, if applicable, for applicants seeking vendorization as community-based day programs;

    (e). The proposed or existing staff qualifications and duty statements as required in Sections 56722 and 56724 of these regulations for applicants seeking vendorization as community-based day programs;

(f). The proposed or existing service design as required in Section 56780 of these regulations for applicants seeking vendorization as in-home respite service agencies;

(g). The proposed or existing staff qualifications and duty statements as required in Sections 56790 and 56792 of these regulations for applicants seeking vendorization as in-home respite services agencies;

(h). The proposed service design as required in Sections 58630 and 58631 of these regulations for applicants seeking vendorization to provide supported living service;

(i). The signed agreement with the Department of Health Services, Form DS 1896, dated 12/93, entitled Medi-Cal Program Provider Agreement Claim Certification, obtainable from the regional centers as part of the vendorization packet, for those applicants whose proposed service is eligible for Medi-Cal reimbursement; and

(j). The proposed program design as required by Subchapter 4.1, Section 56084 for those applicants seeking vendorization.

(k). The applicant shall sign and date Form DS 1890 (12/92), which includes a certification that the information is true, correct and complies with Title 17, Section 54310(a).

(l). In addition to subsection (a). the vendor shall specify the following information: The name, title, business address and telephone number of each officer and member of the governing board;

The application shall include copies of the corporation's articles of incorporation; by-laws, which shall include provisions for control by a responsible governing board; annual statement filed with the Secretary of State; corporate charter, if applicable; and evidence certifying the corporation's nonprofit status.

The application shall contain a written resolution from the governing board stating that the board shall operate the facility in conformity with all applicable statutes and regulations.

Disclosure of:

1. Any board member's or officer's prior or present service as an administrator, general partner, corporate officer or director of any health facility certified by the Department of Health Services or community care facility licensed by the Department of Social Services' Community Care Licensing Division; and

2. Any revocation or other action taken, or in the process of being taken, against any community care facility license or health facility certification held or previously held by the applicant or any officer or member of the governing board.

3. A financial statement and budget which demonstrate the applicant's ability to pay for the costs of operating the facility to provide the level of services and supports necessary to maintain consumers for whom the Regional Center is responsible for;

4. A written statement that the facility shall be approved by the community care licensing office as a residence for a consumer.

5. Any other information required by the regional center which is pertinent to vendorization of the facility.

Step 12: Community Care Licensing Representative to visit the facility to confirm compliance with the regulation (Third Stage / Component).

- Placement agency representative to visit the facility.
- Review of Application: Ninety (90) Day Review
- Return application for revision, approval or denial. If correction is required, the applicant must respond within 30 days from date of notice of correction.
- Second Visit from Community Care Facility representative LPA
- Second visit from placement agencies (optional)

HERE ARE SOME IMPORTANT TIPS TO OBSERVE WHEN YOUR FACILITY IS SCHEDULED FOR INITIAL LPA VISIT:

a. Fire marshal certificate of occupancy

b. Safety, cleanliness and orderliness of the facility.

c. The home and its furnishings in excellent livable condition

d. Heating and Air-conditioning must be in good working condition.

e. Food supplies to accommodate in case of full capacity occupancy.

f. Operations manual

g. Medications and chemical supplies

h. Beds and furniture in excellent condition.

i. Fire and safety precautions

j. Emergency plan

k. Windows, doors, cabinets, etc.. must be in functioning order

l. Over-all condition of the facility must meet all public agency and regulation standards for safety.

Step 13: Approval of License to Operate. Issuance of Provisional License (if no pending major issues on the application).

Upon visit of the facility by the LPA and when based on reports and recommendations by the LPA the facility meets the standards provided under the state and federal regulations and no pending major issues/requirements, the facility may be issued temporary license to operate which is normally valid for at least six months or up to one year if there are some minor insignificant issues. Upon completion of all requirements, provisional license may be renewed and adjusted to one year depending on the past and succeeding facility performance in meeting the expectations and guidelines under the regulations.

Step 14: Business Officially Begins upon receipt of a provisional license to operate.

Provisional license is normally issued to brand new applicants who meet the requirements. Provisional license is normally good for at least six months and if the business remains in excellent to good standing with Community Care Licensing. Upon renewal the license is converted into permanent license which is valid for one a year or more depending on operation.

Clients referred to the applicant's facility as the adventure BEGINS.

EXHIBIT ONE:
(Sample Articles of Incorporation Form)

Corporation Name

Article One
Corporate Name

The name of the corporation is _____
                                    Corporation Name

Article Two
Purpose

The purpose of the corporation is to engage in any lawful act or activity for which a corporation may be organized under the General Corporation Law of California other than the banking, the trust company business or the practice of a profession permitted to be incorporated by the California Corporations Code.

Article Three
Registered Office/Agent

The name and address in the State of California of this corporation's initial agent for service of process is:

Name: _____
Address: _____, City _____ State ___ Zip: ___

Article Four
Initial Officers

Names and addresses of persons who are appointed to act as the initial directors of this corporation are:

Name: _____ Director   Name: _____ Director

Name: _____ Director   Name: _____ Director

Article Five
Authorized Capital Stock

The corporation is authorized to issue only one class of shares of stock; and the total number of shares which the corporation is authorized to issue is _____
(Indicate how many stocks)

Signatures:

Name: _____ Director

Name: _____ Director

Romwell Martinez Sabeniano, MBA.HCM

We declare that we are the persons who executed the foregoing Articles of Incorporation which execution is our act and deed.

Signatures:

_____
Name: **Director**

_____
Name: **Director**

Mail a copy to: **Secretary of State**
State of California
Business Programs
Legal Review Unit
1500 – 11th Street
Sacramento, Ca. 95814

You can also register on-line thru the internet by logging in to the Secretary of State Website located at: ww.ss.ca.gov

An Easy Guide On How to Establish Your First Residential Care Facility

(Sample By-Laws)

BY LAWS

OF

CHILDREN OF UNCLE SAM FOUNDATION

(A California Non-Profit Corporation)

ARTICLE ONE

OFFICES

Section 1. Principal Office: The principal office of the corporation for the transaction of its business is located at _____, _____, Ca. _____

Section 2. Change of Address: The county of the corporation's principal office can be changed only by amendment of these By-Laws and not otherwise. The Board of Directors may, however, change the principal office from one location to another within the named county by noting the changed address and effective date below, and such changes of address shall not be deemed an amendment of these By-Laws:

_____ Dated _____
Signed:

_____ Dated: _____
Signed:

_____ Dated: _____
Signed:

Section 3. Other Offices: The corporation may also have offices at such other places, within or outside the State of California where it is qualified to do business, as its business may require and as the board of Directors may, from time to time, designate.

ARTICLE TWO

PURPOSES

Section 1. Objectives and Purposes: As a non-profit organization, our mission is to help uplift the life and condition of abused and neglected children by providing a high quality service and residential care facility available 24 hours to service the needs of these children.

The primary objectives and purposes of this corporation shall be: To establish an organization that will create and provide a residential care facility for children who are under the juvenile court system where they will be given the love and nurturing they deserve as well as to teach them the basic knowledge and skills that they need in order to be able to cope with the challenges of the society.

To acquire a facility where the organization can conduct seminars, training and provide personalized service and or training to private individuals, groups or corporations who wants to learn how to care and assist these children with special needs.

ARTICLE THREE

DIRECTORS

Section 1. Number: The corporation shall have FOUR DIRECTORS and collectively they shall be known as the Board of Directors. The number may be changed by amendment of this By-Laws, or by repeal of this By-Law and adoption of a new By- law, as provided in these By-Laws.

Section 2. Power: Subject to the provisions of the California Non-Profit Benefit Corporation law and any limitations in the Articles of Incorporation and By-Laws relating to action required or permitted to be taken or approved by the members, if any, of this corporation, the activities and affairs of this corporation shall be conducted and all corporate powers shall be exercised by or under the direction of the Board of Directors.

Section 3. Duties: It shall be the duty of the Directors to:

   (a). Perform any and all duties imposed on them collectively or individually by law, the Articles of Incorporation of this corporation, or by these By-Laws;

   (b). Appoint and remove, employ and discharge, and except as otherwise provided in these By-Laws, prescribe the duties and affix the compensation, if any, of all officers, agents and employees of the corporation;

   (c). Supervise all officers, agents and employees of the corporation to assure that their duties are performed properly;

   (d). Meet at such times and places as required by these By-laws;

   (e). Register their addresses with the Secretary of the corporation and notices of meetings mailed or telegraphed to them at such addressed shall be valid notices thereof.

Section 4. Terms of Office: Each Director shall hold office until the next annual meeting for election of the Board of Directors as specified in this By-Laws, and until his or her successor is elected and qualifies.

Section 5. Compensation: Directors shall serve without compensation or payment. Directors may not be compensated for rendering services to the corporation in any capacity other than director unless such other compensation is reasonable and is allowable under the provisions of Section 6 of this article.

Section 6. Restriction Regarding Interested Directors.:
Notwithstanding any other provision of these By-Laws, not more than forty nine percent (49%) of the persons serving on the board may be interested persons. For purposes of this Section, "interested persons" mean either:

   (a). Any person currently being compensated by the corporation for services rendered if within the previous twelve (12) months, whether as a full-or part-time officer or other employee, independent contractor, or otherwise, excluding any reasonable compensation paid to a director as director; or

(b). Any brother, sister, ancestor, or descendant, spouse, brother-in-law, sister-in-law, son-in-law, daughter-in-law, mother-in-law, or father-in-law of any such person.

Section 7. Place of Meetings: Meetings shall be held at the principal office of the corporation unless otherwise provided by the board or at such place within or without the State of California which has been designated from time to time by resolution of the Board of Directors. In the absence of such designation, any meeting not held at the principal office of the corporation shall be valid only if held on the written consent of all directors given either before or after the meeting and filed with the Secretary of the corporation or after all board members have been given written notice of the meeting as hereinafter provided for special meetings of the board. Any meetings, regular or special, may be held by conference telephone or similar communications equipment, so as long as all directors participating in such meeting can hear one another.

Section 8. Regular and Annual Meetings: Regular meetings of Directors shall be held on first Friday of January at 10:00AM, unless such day falls on a legal holiday, in which event the regular meetings shall be held at the same hour and place on the next business day.

If this corporation makes no provision for members, then, at the annual meeting of directors held on First Friday of January, directors shall be elected by the Board of Directors in accordance with this section. Cumulative voting by directors for the election of directors shall not be permitted. The candidates receiving the highest number of votes up to the number of directors to be elected shall be elected. Each director shall cast one vote with voting being by ballot only.

Section 9. Special Meetings: Special meetings of the Board of Directors may be called by the Chairperson of the board, the President, the Vice President, the Secretary, or by any two directors and such meetings shall be held at the place, within or without the

State of California, designated by the person or persons calling the meeting, and in the absence of such designation, at the principal office of the corporation.

Section 10. Notice of Meetings: Regular meetings of the board may be held without notice. Special meetings of the board shall be held upon four (4) days' notice by first-class mail or forty-eight (48) hours' notice delivered personally or by telephone or telegraph. If sent by mail or telegraph, the notice shall be deemed to be delivered on its deposit in the mails or on its delivery to the telegraph company. Such notices shall be addressed to each director at his or her address as shown on the books of the corporation. Notice of the time and place of holding an adjourned meeting need not be given to absent directors if the time and place of the adjourned meeting are fixed at the meeting adjourned and if such adjourned meeting is held no more than twenty-four (24) hours from the time of the original meeting. Notice shall be given of any adjourned regular or special meetings to directors absent from the original meeting is held more than twenty-four (24) hours from the time of the original meeting.

Section 11. Contents of Notice: Notice of meetings not herein dispensed with shall specify the place, day and hour of the meeting. The purpose of any board meeting need not be specified in the notice.

Section 12. Waiver of Notice and Consent to Holding Meetings: The transactions of any meetings of the board, however called and noticed or wherever held, are as valid as though the meeting had been duly held after proper call and notice, provided a quorum, as hereinafter defined, is present and provided that either before or after the meeting each director not present signs a waiver of notice, a consent to holding the meeting, or an approval of the minutes thereof. All such waivers, consents, or approvals shall be filed with the corporate records or made a part for the minutes of the meeting.

Section 13. Quorum for Meetings: A quorum shall consist of Three or all of the Four Directors. Except as otherwise provided in these Bylaws or in the Articles of Incorporation of this corporation, or by law, no business shall be considered by the board at any meetings at which a quorum, as hereinafter defined, is not present, and the one motion which the Chair shall entertain at such meeting is a motion to adjourn. However, a majority of the directors present at such meeting may adjourn from time to time until the time fixed for the next regular meeting of the board.

When the meeting is adjourned for lack of quorum, it shall not be necessary to give any notice of the time and place of the adjourned meeting or of the business to be transacted at such meeting, other than by announcement at the meeting at which the adjournment is taken, except as provided in Section 10 of this Article.

The directors present at a duly called and held meeting at which a quorum is initially present may continue to do business notwithstanding the loss of a quorum at the meeting due to a withdrawal of directors from the meeting, provided that any action thereafter taken must be approved by at least a majority of the required quorum for such meeting, or such greater percentage as may be required by law, or the Articles of Incorporation or Bylaws of this corporation.

Section 14. Majority Action as Board Action: Every act or decision done or made by a majority of the directors present at a meeting duly held at which a quorum is present is the act of the Board of Directors, unless the Articles of Incorporation or Bylaws of this corporation, or provisions of the California Nonprofit Public Benefit Corporation Law, particularly those provisions relating to appointment of committees (Section 5212), approval of contracts or transactions in which a director has a material financial interest (Section 5233) and indemnification of directors (Section 5238e), require a greater percentage or different voting rules for approval of a matter by the board.

Section 15. Conduct of Meetings: Meetings of the Board of directors shall be presided by the Chairperson of the Board, or, if no such person has been so designated or, in his or her absence, the President of the corporation or, in his or her absence, by the Vice President of the corporation or, in the absence of each of these persons, by a Chairperson chosen by a majority of the directors present at the meeting. The Secretary of the corporation shall act as secretary of all meetings of the board, provided that, in his or her absence, the presiding officer shall appoint another person to act as Secretary of the Meeting.

Meetings shall be governed by rules of procedure, as such rules may be revised from time to time, insofar as such rules are not inconsistent with or in conflict with these Bylaws, with the Articles of Incorporation of this corporation, or with provisions of law.

Section 16. Action By Unanimous Written Consent Without Meeting: Any action required or permitted to be taken by the Board of Directors under any provision of law may be taken without a meeting, if all members of the board shall individually or collectively consent in writing to such action. For the purposes of this Section only, "all members of the board" shall not include any "interested director" as defined in Section 5233 of the California Nonprofit Public Benefit Corporation Law. Such written consent or consents shall be filed with the minutes of the proceedings of the board. Such action by written consent shall have the same force and effect as the unanimous vote of the directors. Any certificate or other document filed under any provision of law which relates to action so taken shall state that the action was taken by unanimous written consent of the Board of Directors without a meeting and that the Bylaws of this corporation authorize the directors to so act, and such statement shall be prima facie evidence of such authority.

Section 17. Vacancies: Vacancies on the Board of Directors shall exist (1) on the death, resignation or removal of any director, and (2) whenever the number of authorized directors is increased.

The Board of Directors may declare vacant the office of a director who has been declared of unsound mind by a final order of court, or convicted of a felony, or been found by a final order or judgment of any court to have breached any duty under Section 5230 and following of the California Nonprofit Public Benefit Corporation Law.

If this corporation has any members, then, if the corporation has less than fifty (50) members, directors may be removed without cause by a majority of all members, or, if the corporation has fifty (50) or more members, by vote of a majority of the votes represented at a membership meeting at which quorum is present.

If this corporation has no members, directors may be removed without cause by a majority of the directors then in office.

Any director may resign effective upon giving written notice to the Chairperson of the Board, the President, the Secretary, or the Board of Directors, unless the notice specifies a later time for the effectiveness of such resignation. No director may resign if the corporation would then be left without a duly elected director or directors in charge of its affairs, except upon notice to the Attorney General.

Vacancies on the board may be filled by approval of the board, or, if the number of directors then in office is less than a quorum, by (1) the unanimous written consent of the directors then in office, (2) the affirmative vote of a majority of the directors then in office at a meeting held pursuant to notice or waivers of notice complying with this Article of these Bylaws, or (3) a sole remaining director. If this corporation has members, however, vacancies created by the removal of the a director may be filled only by the approval of the members. The members, if any, of this corporation may elect a director at any time to fill any vacancy not filled by the directors.

A person elected to fill a vacancy as provided by this Section shall hold office until the next annual election of the Board of Directors or until his or her death, resignation or removal from office.

Section 18. Non-Liability of Directors: The directors shall not be personally liable for the debts, liabilities, or other obligations of the corporation.

Section 19. Indemnification By Corporation Of Directors, Officers, Employees and Other Agents: To the extent that a person who is, or was, a director, officer, employee or other agents of this corporation has been successful on the merits in defense of any civil, criminal, administrative or investigative proceeding brought to procure a judgment against such person by reason of the fact that he or she is, or was, an agent of the corporation, or has been successful in defense of any claim, issue or matter therein, such person shall be indemnified against expenses actually and reasonably incurred by the person in connection with such proceeding.

If such person either settles any such claim or sustains a judgment against him or her, then indemnification against expenses, judgments, fines, settlements and other amounts reasonably incurred in connection with such proceedings shall be provided by this corporation but only to the extent allowed by, and in accordance with the requirements of Section 5238 of the California Nonprofit Public Benefit Corporation Law.

Section 20. Insurance For Corporate Agents: The Board of Directors may adopt a resolution authorizing the purchase and maintenance of insurance on behalf of any agent of the corporation (including a director, officer, employee or other agent of the corporation) against any liability other than for violating provisions of law relating to self-dealing (Section 5233 of the California Nonprofit Public Benefit Corporation Law) asserted against or incurred by the agent in such capacity or arising out of the agent's status as such, whether or not the corporation would have the power to indemnify the agent against such liability under the provisions of Section 5238 of the California Nonprofit Public Benefit Corporation Law.

ARTICLE 4

OFFICERS

Section 1. Number of Officers: The officers of the corporation shall be a President, a Secretary, and a Chief Financial Officer who shall be designated the Treasurer. The corporation may also have, as determined by the Board of Directors, a Chairperson of the Board, one or more Vice Presidents, Assistant Secretaries, Assistant Treasurers, or other officers. Any number of offices may be held by the same person except that neither the Secretary nor the Treasurer may serve as the President or Chairperson of the Board.

Section 2. Qualification, Election, And Term Of Office: Any person may serve as officer of this corporation. Officers shall be elected by the Board of Directors, at any time, and each officer shall hold office until he or she resigns or is removed or is otherwise disqualified to serve, or until his or her successor shall be elected and qualified, whichever occurs first.

Section 3. Subordinate Officers: The Board of Directors may appoint such other officers or agents as it may deem desirable, and such officers shall serve such terms, have such authority, and perform such duties as may be prescribed from time to time by the Board of Directors.

Section 4. Removal and Resignation: Any officer may be removed, either with or without cause, by the Board of Directors, at any time. Any officer may resign at any time by giving written notice to the Board of Directors or to the President or Secretary of the corporation. Any such resignation shall take effect at the date of receipt of such notice or at any later date specified therein, and, unless otherwise specified therein, the acceptance of such resignation shall not be necessary to make it effective. The above provisions of this Section shall be superseded by any conflicting terms of a contract which has been approved or ratified by the Board of Directors relating to the employment of any officer of the corporation.

Section 5. Vacancies: Any vacancy caused by the death, resignation, removal, disqualification, or otherwise, of any officer shall be filled by the Board of Directors. In the event of a vacancy in any officer other than that of President, such vacancy may be filled temporarily by appointment by the President until such time as the Board shall fill the vacancy. Vacancies occurring in offices of officers appointed at the discretion of the board may or may not be filled as the board shall determine.

Section 6. Duties of President: The President shall be the chief executive officer of the corporation and shall, subject to the control of the Board of Directors, supervise and control the affairs of the corporation and the activities of the officers. He or she shall perform all duties incident to his or her office and such other duties as may be required by law, by the articles of Incorporation of this corporation, or by these Bylaws, or which may be prescribed from time to time by the Board of Directors. Unless another person is specifically appointed as Chairperson of the Board of Directors, he or she shall preside at all meetings of the Board of Directors. If applicable, the President shall preside at all meetings of the members. Except as otherwise expressly provided by law, by the Articles of Incorporation, or by these Bylaws, he or she shall, in the name of the corporation, execute such deeds, mortgages, bonds, contracts, checks, or other instruments which may from time to time be authorized by the Board of Directors.

Section 7. Duties of Vice President: In the absence of the President, or in the event of his or her inability or refusal to act, the Vice President shall perform all the duties of the President, and when so acting shall have all the powers of, and be subject to all the restrictions on, the President. the Vice President shall have other powers and perform such other duties as may be prescribed by law, by the Articles of Incorporation, or by these Bylaws, or as may be prescribed by the Board of Directors.

Section 8. Duties of Secretary: The Secretary shall: Certify and keep at the principal office of the corporation the original, or a copy of these Bylaws as amended or otherwise altered to date.

Keep at the principal office of the corporation or at such other place as the board may determine, a book of minutes of all meetings of the directors, and, if applicable, meetings of committees of directors and of members, recording therein the time and place of holding, whether regular or special, how called, how notice thereof was given, the names of those present or represented at the meeting, and the proceedings thereof.

See that all notices are duly given in accordance with the provisions of these Bylaws or as required by law.

Be custodian of the records and of the seal of the corporation and see that the seal is affixed to all duly executed documents, the execution of which on behalf of the corporation under its seal is authorized by law or these Bylaws.

Keep at the principal office of the corporation a membership book containing the name and address of each and any members, and, in the case where any membership has been terminated, he or she shall record such fact in the membership book together with the date on which such membership ceased.

Exhibit at all reasonable times to any director of the corporation, or to his or her agent or attorney on request therefore, the Bylaws, the membership book, and the minutes of the proceedings of the directors of the corporation.

In general, perform all duties incident to the office of Secretary and such other duties as may be required by law, by the Articles of Incorporation of this corporation, or by these Bylaws, or which may be assigned to him or her from time to time by the Board of Directors.

Section 9. Duties of Treasurer: Subject to the provisions of these Bylaws relating to the "Execution of Instruments, Deposits and Funds," the Treasurer shall:

Have charge and custody of, and be responsible for, all funds and securities of the corporation, and deposit all such funds in the name of the corporation in such banks, trust companies, or other depositories as shall be selected by the Board of Directors.

Receive, and give receipt for, moneys due and payable to the corporation from any source whatsoever.

Disburse, or cause to be disbursed, the funds of the corporation as may be directed by the Board of Directors, taking proper vouchers for such disbursements.

Keep and maintain adequate and correct accounts of the corporation's properties and business transactions, including accounts of its assets, liabilities, receipts, disbursements, gains and losses.

Exhibit at all reasonable times the books of account and financial records to any director of the corporation, or to his or her agent or attorney, on request therefore.

Render to the president and directors, whenever requested, an account of any or all of his or her transactions as Treasurer and of the financial condition of the corporation.

Prepare, or cause to be prepared, and certify, or cause to be certified, the financial statements to be included in any requested reports.

In general, perform all duties incident to the office of Treasurer and such offer duties as may be required by law, by the Articles of Incorporation of the corporation, or by these Bylaws, or which may be assigned to him or her from time to time by the Board of Directors.

Section 10. Compensation: The salaries of the officers, if any, shall be fixed from time to time by resolution of the Board of Directors, and no officer shall be prevented from receiving such salary by reason of the fact that he or she is also a director of the corporation, provided, however, that such compensation paid a director for serving as an officer of this corporation shall only be allowed if permitted under the provisions of Article 3, Section 6 of these Bylaws. In all cases, any salaries received by officers of this corporation shall be reasonable and given in return for services actually rendered for the corporation which relate to the performance of the charitable or public purposes of this corporation.

ARTICLE 5

COMMITTEES

Section 1. Executive Committee: The Board of Directors may, by a majority vote of directors, designate two (2) or more of its members (who may also be serving as officers of this corporation) to constitute an Executive Committee and delegate to such Committee any powers and authority of the board in the management of the business and affairs of the corporation, except with respect to:

- (a). The approval of any action which, under law or the provisions of these Bylaws, requires the approval of the members or of a majority of all the members.

- (b). The filling of vacancies on the board or on any committee which has the authority of the board.

- (c). The fixing of compensation of the directors for serving on the board or any committee.

(d). The amendment or repeal of Bylaws or the adoption of new Bylaws.

(e). The amendment or repeal of any resolution of the board which by its express terms is not so amenable or repealable.

(f). The appointment of committees of the board or the members thereof.

(g). The expenditure of corporate funds to support a nominee for director after there are more people nominated for director than can be elected.

(h). The approval of any transaction to which this corporation is a party and in which one or more of the directors has a material financial interest, except as expressly provided in Section 5233 (d) (3) of the California Nonprofit Public Benefit Corporation Law.

By a majority vote of its members then in office, the board may at any time revoke or modify any or all of the authority so delegated, increase or decrease but not below two (2) the number of its members, and fill vacancies therein from the members of the board. The Committee shall keep regular minutes of its proceedings, cause them to be filed with the corporate records, and report the same to the board from time to time as the board may require.

Section 2. Other Committees: The corporation shall have such other committees as may from time to time be designated by resolution of the Board of Directors. such other committees may consist of persons who are not also members of the board. These additional committees shall act in an advisory capacity only to the board and shall be clearly titled as "advisory" committees.

Section 3. Meetings and Action of Committees: Meetings and action of committees shall be governed by, noticed, held and taken in accordance with the provisions of these Bylaws concerning meetings of the Board of Directors, with such changes in the context of such Bylaw provisions as are necessary to substitute the committee and its members for the Board of Directors and its members, except that the time for regular meetings of committees may be fixed by resolution of the Board of Directors. The Board of Directors may also adopt rules and regulations pertaining to the conduct of meetings of committees to the extent that such rules and regulations are not inconsistent with the provisions of these Bylaws.

ARTICLE 6

EXECUTION OF INSTRUMENTS, DEPOSITS AND FUNDS

Section 1. Execution of Instruments: The Board of Directors, except as otherwise provided in these By-Laws, may by resolution authorize any officer or agent of the corporation to enter into any contract or execute and deliver any instrument in the name of and on behalf of the corporation, and such authority may be general or confined to specific instances. Unless so authorized, no officer, agent, or employee shall have any power or authority to bind the corporation by any contract or engagement or to pledge its credit or to render it liable monetarily for any purpose in any amount.

Section 2. Checks and Notes: Except as otherwise specifically determined by resolution of the Board of Directors, or as otherwise required by law, checks, drafts, promissory notes, orders for the payment of money, and other evidence of indebtedness of the corporation shall be signed by the Treasurer and countersigned by the President of the Corporation.

Section 3. Deposits: All funds of the corporation shall be deposited from time to time to the credit of the corporation in such banks, trust companies, or other depositories as the Board of Directors may select.

Section 4. Gifts: The Board of Directors may accept on behalf of the corporation any contribution, gift, bequest, or devise for the charitable or public purposes of this corporation.

ARTICLE 7

CORPORATE RECORDS, REPORTS AND SEAL

Section 1. Maintenance of Corporate Records: The corporation shall keep at its principal office in the State of California:

(a). Minutes of all meetings of directors, committees of the board, and, if this corporation has members, of all meetings of members, indicating the time and place of holding such meetings, whether regular or special, how called, the notice given, and the names of those present and the proceedings thereof;

(b). Adequate and correct books and records of account, including accounts of its properties and business transactions and accounts of its assets, liabilities, receipts, disbursements, gains and

(c). A record of its members, if any, indicating their names and addresses and, if applicable, the class of membership held by each member and the termination date of any membership;

(d). A copy of the corporation's Articles of Incorporation and Bylaws as amended to date, which shall be open to inspection by members, if any, of the corporation at all reasonable times during office hours.

Section 2.. Corporate Seal: The Board of Directors may adopt, use, and at will alter, a corporate seal. Such seal shall be kept at the principal office of the corporation. Failure to affix the seal to corporate instruments, however, shall not affect the validity of any such instrument.

Section 3. Directions Inspection Rights: Every director shall have the absolute right at any reasonable time to inspect and copy all books, records and documents of every kind and to inspect the physical properties of the corporation.

Section 4. Members' Inspection Rights: If this corporation has any members, then each and every member shall have the following inspection rights, for a purpose reasonably related to the person's interest as a member:

(a) To inspect and copy the record of all members' names, addresses and voting rights at reasonable times, upon five (5) business days' prior written demand on the corporation, which demand shall state the purpose for which the inspection rights are requested.

(b). To obtain from the Secretary of the corporation, upon written demand and payment of a reasonable charge, an alphabetized list of the names, addresses and voting rights of those members entitled to vote for the election of the directors as of the most recent record date for which the list has been compiled or as of the date specified by the member subsequent to the date of demand. The demand shall state the purpose for which the list is requested. The membership list shall be made available on or before the later of ten (10) business days after the demand is received or after the date specified therein as of which the list is to be compiled.

(c). To inspect at any reasonable time the books, records, or minutes of proceedings of the members or of the board or committees of the board, upon written demand on the corporation by the members, for a purpose reasonably related to such person's interest as a member.

Section 5. Rights To Copy and Make Extracts: Any inspection under the provisions of this Article may be made in person or by agent or attorney and the right to inspection includes the right to copy and make extracts.

Section 6. Annual Report: The board shall cause an annual report to be furnished not later than one hundred and twenty (120) days after the close of the corporation's fiscal year to all directors of the corporation and, if this corporation has members, to any member who request it in writing, which report shall contain the following information in appropriate detail.

- (a). The assets and liabilities, including the trust funds, of the corporation as of the end of the fiscal year;

- (b). The principal changes in assets and liabilities, including trust funds, during the fiscal year;

- (c). The revenue or receipts of the corporation, both unrestricted and restricted to particular purposes, for the fiscal year;

- (d). The expenses or disbursements of the corporation, for both general and restricted purposes, during the fiscal year;

- (e). Any information required by Section 7 of this Article.

The annual report shall be accompanied by any report thereon of independent accountants, or, if there is no such report the certificate of an authorized officer of the corporation that such statements were prepared without audit from the books and records of the corporation.

If this corporation has members, then, if this corporation receives TWENTY-FIVE THOUSAND DOLLARS ($25,000), or more, in gross revenues or receipts during the fiscal year, this corporation shall automatically send the above annual report to all members, in such manner, at such time, and with such contents, including an accompanying report from independent accountants or certification of a corporate officer, as specified by the above provisions of this Section relating to the annual report.

Section 7. Annual Statement of Specific Transactions to Members: This corporation shall mail or deliver to all directors and any and all members a statement within one hundred and twenty (120) days after the close of its fiscal year which briefly describe the amount and circumstances of any indemnification or transaction of the following kind:

(a). Any transaction in which the corporation, or its parent or its subsidiary, was a party, and in which either of the following had a direct or indirect material financial interest:

(b). Any director or officer of the corporation, or its parent or subsidiary (a mere common directorship shall not be considered a material financial interest); or

(c). Any holder of more than ten percent (10%) of the voting power of the corporation, its parent or its subsidiary.

The above statement need only be provided with respect to a transaction during the previous fiscal year involving more than FIFTY THOUSAND DOLLARS ($50,000) or which as one of a number of transactions with the same persons involving, in the aggregate, more than FIFTY THOUSAND DOLLARS ($50,000).

Similarly, the statement need only be provided with respect to indemnification or advances aggregating more than TEN THOUSAND DOLLARS ($10,000) paid during the previous fiscal year to any director or officer, except that no such statement need be made if such indemnification was approved by the members pursuant to Section 5238 (e) (2) of the California Nonprofit Public Benefit Corporation Law.

Any statement required by the Section shall briefly describe the names of the interested persons involved in such transactions, stating each person's relationship to the corporation, the nature of such person's interest in the transaction and, where practical, the amount of such interest, provided that in the case of a transaction with a partnership of which such person is a partner, only the interest of the partnership need be stated.

If this corporation has any members and provides all members with an annual report according to the provisions of Section 6 of this Article, then such annual report shall include the information required by this Section.

ARTICLE 8

FISCAL YEAR

Section 1. Fiscal Year of the Corporation: The fiscal year of the corporation shall begin on the 1st day of January and end on the 31st day of December in each year.

ARTICLE 9

AMENDMENT OF BYLAWS

Section 1. Amendment: Subject to any provision of law applicable to the amendment of Bylaws of public benefit nonprofit corporations, these Bylaws, or any of them, may be altered, amended, or repealed and new Bylaws adopted as follows:

(a). Subject to the power of members, if any, to change or repeal these Bylaws under Section 5150 of the Corporations Code, by approval of the Board of Directors unless the Bylaw amendment would materially and adversely affect the rights of members, if any, as to voting or transfer, provided, however, if this corporation has admitted any members, then a Bylaw specifying or changing the fixed number of directors of the corporation, the maximum or minimum number of directors, or changing from a fixed to variable board or vice versa, may not be adopted, amended, or repealed except as provided in subparagraph (b) of this Section; or

(b). By approval of the members, if any, of this corporation.

ARTICLE 10

AMENDMENT OF ARTICLES

Section 1. Amendment of Articles Before Admission of Members: Before any members have been admitted to the corporation, any amendment of the Articles of Incorporation may be adopted by approval of the Board of Directors.

Section 2. Amendment of Articles After Admission of Members: After members, if any, have been admitted to the corporation, amendment of the Articles of Incorporation may be adopted by approval of the Board of Directors and by the approval of the members of this corporation.

Section 3. Certain Amendments: Notwithstanding the above Sections of this Article, this corporation shall not amend its Articles of Incorporation to alter any statement which appears in the original Articles of Incorporation of the names and addresses of the first directors of this corporation, nor the name and address of its initial agent, except to correct an error in such statement or to delete such statement after the corporation has filed a "Statement by a Domestic Non-Profit Corporation" pursuant to Section 6210 of the California Nonprofit Corporation Law.

ARTICLE 11

PROHIBITION AGAINST SHARING CORPORATE PROFITS AND ASSETS

Section 1. Prohibition Against Sharing Corporate Profits and Assets. No member, director, officer, employee, or other person connected with this corporation, or any private individual, shall receive at any time any of the net earnings or pecuniary profit from the operations of the corporation, provided, however, that this provision shall not prevent payment to any such person of reasonable compensation for services performed for the corporation in effecting any of its public or charitable purposes, provided that such compensation is otherwise permitted by these Bylaws and is fixed by resolution of the Board of Directors; and no such person or persons shall be entitled to share in the distribution of, and shall not receive, any of the corporate assets on dissolution of the corporation. All members, if any, of the corporation shall be deemed to have expressly consented and agreed that no such dissolution or winding up of the affairs of the corporation, whether voluntarily or involuntarily, the assets of the corporation, after all debts have been satisfied, shall be distributed as required by the Articles of Incorporation of this corporation and not otherwise.

ARTICLE 12

MEMBERS

Section 1. Determination of Members. If this corporation makes no provision for members, then, pursuant to Section 5310 (b) of the Nonprofit Public Benefit Corporation Law of the State of California, any action which would otherwise, under law or the provisions of the Articles of Incorporation or Bylaws of this corporation, require approval by a majority of all members or approval by the members, shall only require the approval of the Board of Directors.

WRITTEN CONSENT OF DIRECTORS ADOPTING BYLAWS

We, the undersigned, are all of the persons named as the initial directors in the Articles of Incorporation of Children of Uncle Sam Foundation, a California nonprofit corporation, and, pursuant to the authority granted to the directors by these Bylaws to take action by unanimous written consent without meeting, consent, consent to, and hereby do, adopt the foregoing Bylaws, consisting of _____ pages, as the Bylaws of this corporation.

_____   _____
Director   Director

                                     Dated: _____
_____
Director

CERTIFICATE

This is to certify that the foregoing is a true and correct copy of the Bylaws of the corporation named in the title thereto and that such Bylaws were duly adopted by the Board of Directors of said corporation.

Dated:_____

_____
Secretary

ARTICLE 12

MEMBERS

Section 1. Determination and Rights of Members: The corporation shall have only one class of members. No member shall hold more than one membership in the corporation. Except as expressly provided in or authorized by the Articles of Incorporation or Bylaws of this corporation, all memberships shall have the same rights, privileges, restrictions and conditions.

Section 2.. Qualifications of Members: The is no qualification requirement to become a member in this corporation.

Section 3. Admission of Members: Applicants shall be admitted to membership regardless of age, race, color, creed, nationality or religion.

Section 4. Fees, Dues, and Assessments: There shall be no fee for membership in the corporation:

Section 5. Number of Members. There is no limit on the number of members the corporation may admit.

Section 6. Membership Book. The corporation shall keep a membership book containing the name and address of each member. Termination of the membership of any member shall be recorded in the book, together with the date of termination of such membership. Such book shall be kept at the corporations principal office and shall be available for inspection by any director or member of the corporation during regular business hours.

The record of names and addresses of the members of this corporation shall constitute the membership list of this corporation and shall not be used in, in whole or part, by any person for any purpose not reasonably related to a member's interest as a member.

Section 7. Non-Liability of Members. A member of this corporation is not, as such, personally liable for the debts, liabilities, or obligations of the corporation.

Section 8. Non-Transferability of Memberships. No member may transfer a membership or any right arising there from. All rights of membership cease upon the member's death.

Section 9. Termination of Membership
(a). Grounds of Termination. The membership of a member shall terminate upon the occurrence of any of the following events:

    (1). Upon his or her notice of such termination delivered to the President of Secretary of the corporation personally or by mail, such membership to terminate upon the date of delivery of the notice or date of deposit in the mail.

    (2). Upon a determination by the Board of Directors that the member has engaged in conduct materially and seriously prejudicial to the interests or purposes of the corporation.

    (3). If this corporation has provided for the payment of dues by members, upon a failure to renew his or her membership by paying dues on or before their due date, such termination to be effective thirty (30) days after a written notification of delinquency is given personally or mailed to such member by the Secretary of the corporation. A member may avoid such termination by paying the amount of delinquent dues within a thirty (30)-day period following the member's receipt of the written notification of delinquency.

(b). Procedure for Expulsion. Following the determination that a member should be expelled under subparagraph (a) (2) of this section, the following procedure shall be implemented:

    (1). A notice shall be sent by first-class or registered mail to the last address of the member as shown on the corporation's records, setting forth the expulsion and the reasons therefore. Such notice shall be sent at least fifteen (15) days before the proposed effective date of the expulsion.

(2). The member being expelled shall be given opportunity to be heard, either orally or in writing, at a hearing to be held not less than five (5) days before the effective date of the proposed expulsion. The hearing to be held by the Board of Directors in accordance with the quorum and voting rules set forth in these Bylaws applicable to the meetings of the Board. The notice to the member of his or her proposed expulsion shall state the date, time, and place of the hearing on his or her proposed expulsion.

(3). Following the hearing, The Board of Directors shall decide whether or not the member should in fact be expelled, suspended, or sanctioned in some other way. The decision of the Board shall be final.

(4). If this corporation has provided for the payment of dues by members, any person expelled from the corporation shall receive a refund of dues already paid. The refund shall be pro-rated to return only the un-accrued balance remaining for the period of the dues payment.

Section 10. Rights on Termination of Membership. All rights of a member in the corporation shall cease on termination of membership as herein provided.

Section 11. Amendments Resulting in the Termination of Memberships. Notwithstanding any other provision of these Bylaws, if any amendment of the Articles of Incorporation or of the Bylaws of this corporation would result in the termination of all memberships or any class of memberships, then such amendment or amendments shall be effected only in accordance with the provisions of Section 5342 of the California Nonprofit Public Benefit Corporation Law.

ARTICLE 13

MEETINGS OF MEMBERS

Section 1. Place of Meetings. Meetings of members shall be held at the principal office of the corporation or at such other place or places within or without the State of California as may be designated from time to time by resolution of the Board of Directors.

Section 2. Annual and Other Regular Meetings. The members shall meet annually on the first Friday of January in each year, at 10:00 AM, for the purpose of electing directors and transacting other business as may come before the meeting. Cumulative voting for the election of directors shall not be permitted. The candidates receiving the highest number of votes up to the number of directors to be elected shall be elected. Each voting member shall cast one vote, with voting being by ballot only. The annual meeting of members for the purposes of electing directors shall be deemed a regular meeting and any reference in these Bylaws to regular meetings of members refers to this annual meeting.

Other regular meetings of the members shall be held on every six months, at 10AM.

If the day fixed for the annual meeting or other regular meetings falls on a legal holiday, such meetings shall be held at the same hour and place on the next business day.

Section 3. Special Meetings of Members. (a) Persons Who May Call Special Meetings of Members. Special meetings of the members shall be called by the Board of Directors, the Chairperson of the Board, or the President of the corporation. In addition, special meetings of the members for any lawful purpose may be called by five percent (5%) or more of the members.

Section 4. Notice of Meetings. (a). Time of Notice. `Whenever members are required or permitted to take action at a meeting, a written notice of the meeting shall be given by the Secretary of the corporation not less than ten (10) nor more than ninety(90) days before the date of the meeting to each member who, on the record date for the notice of the meeting, is entitled to vote thereat, provided, however, that if notice is given by mail, and the notice is not mailed by first- class, registered, or certified mail, that notice shall be given twenty (20) days before the meeting.

> (b). Manner of Giving Notice. Notice of a members' meeting or any report shall be given either personally or by mail or

other means of written communication, addressed to the member at the address of such member appearing on the books of the corporation or given by the member to the corporation for the purpose of notice; or if no address appears or is given, at the place where the principal office of the corporation is located or by publication of notice of the meeting at least once in a newspaper of general circulation in the county in which the principal office is located. Notice shall be deemed to have been given at a time when delivered personally or deposited in the mail or sent by telegram or other means of written communication.

(c). <u>Contents of Notice.</u> Notice of a membership meeting shall state the place, date, and time of the meeting and (1) in the case of a special meeting, the general nature of the business to be transacted, and no other business may be transacted, or (2) in the case of a regular meeting, those matters which the Board, at the time notice is given, intends to present for action by the members. Subject to any provision to the contrary contained in these Bylaws, however, any proper matter may be presented at a regular meeting, for such action. The notice of any meeting of members at which directors are to be elected shall include the names of all those who are nominees at the time notice is given to members.

(d). <u>Notice of Meetings Called By Members</u>. If a special meeting is called by members as authorized by these Bylaws, the request for the meeting shall be submitted in writing, specifying the general nature of the business proposed to be transacted and shall be delivered personally or sent by registered mail or by telegraph to the Chairperson of the Board, President, Vice President or Secretary of the corporation. The officer receiving the request shall promptly cause notice to be given to the members entitled to vote that a meeting will be held, stating the date of the meeting. The date for such meeting shall be fixed by the Board and shall not be less than thirty-five (35) nor more than ninety (90) days after the receipt of the request for the meeting by the officer. If the notice is not given within twenty (20) days after the receipt of the request, person calling the meeting may give the notice themselves.

(e). <u>Waiver of Notice of Meetings.</u> The transactions of any meetings of members, however called and noticed, and wherever held, shall be as valid as though taken at a meeting duly held after regular call and notice, if a quorum is present either in person or by proxy, and if, either before or after the meeting, each of the persons entitled to vote, not present in person or by proxy, signs a written waiver of notice or a consent to the holding of the meeting or an approval of the minutes thereof. All such waiver's, consents and approvals shall be filed with the corporate records or made a part of the minutes of the meeting. Waiver of notices or consents need not specify either the business to be transacted or the purpose of any regular or special meeting of members, except that if action is taken or proposed to be taken for approval of any of the matters specified in subparagraph (f) of this section, the waiver of notice or consent shall state the general nature of the proposal.

(f). <u>Special Notice Rules for Approving Certain Proposals.</u> If action is proposed to be taken or is taken with respect to the following proposals, such action shall be invalid unless unanimously approved by those entitled to vote or unless the general nature of the proposal is stated in the notice of meeting or in any written waiver of notice:

1. Removal of directors without cause;
2. Filling of vacancies on the Board by members;
3. Amending the Articles of Incorporation; and
4. An election to voluntarily wind up and dissolve the corporation.

Section 5. Quorum for Meetings. A quorum shall consists of majority of the voting members of the corporation.

The members present at a duly called and held meeting at which a quorum is initially present may continue to do business notwithstanding the loss of a quorum at the meeting due to a withdrawal of members from the meeting provided that any action taken after the loss of a quorum must be approved by at least a majority of the members required to constitute a quorum.

In the absence of a quorum, any meeting of the members may be adjourned from time to time by the vote of a majority of the votes represented in person or by proxy at the meeting, but no other business shall be transacted at such meeting.

When a meeting is adjourned for lack of sufficient number of members at the meetings or otherwise, it shall not be necessary to give any notice of the time and place of the adjourned meeting of the business to be transacted at such meeting other than by announcement at the meeting at which the adjournment is taken of the time and place of the adjourned meeting. However, if after the adjournment a new record date is fixed for notice or voting, a notice of the adjourned meeting, is entitled to vote at the meeting. A meeting shall not be adjourned for more than forty-five (45) days.

Notwithstanding any other provision of this Article, if this corporation authorizes members to conduct a meeting with a quorum of less than one third (1/3) of the voting power, then, if less than one-third (1/3) of the voting power actually attends a regular meeting, in person or by proxy, then no action may be taken on a matter unless the general nature of the matter was stated in the notice of the regular meeting.

Section 6. Majority Action as Membership Action. Every act or decision done or made by a majority of voting members present in person or by proxy at a duly held meeting at which a quorum is present is the act of the members, unless the law, the Articles of Incorporation of this corporation, or these Bylaws require a greater number.

Section 7. Voting Rights. Each member is entitled to one vote on each matter submitted to a vote by the members. Voting at duly held meetings shall be by voice vote. Election of directors, however, shall be by ballot.

Section 8. Proxy Voting. Members are entitled / permitted to vote or act by proxy. If membership voting by proxy is not allowed by the preceding sentence, no provision in this or other sections of these Bylaws referring to proxy voting shall be construed to permit any member to vote or act by proxy.

If membership voting by proxy is allowed, members entitled to vote shall have the right to vote either in person or by a written proxy executed by such person or by his or her duly authorized agent and filed with the Secretary of the corporation, provided, however, that no proxy shall be valid after eleven (11) months from the date of its execution unless otherwise provided in the proxy. In any case, however, the maximum term of any proxy shall be three (3) years from the date of its execution. No proxy shall be irrevocable and may be revoked following the procedures given in Section 5613 of the California Nonprofit Public Benefit Corporation Law.

If membership voting by proxy is allowed, all proxies shall state general nature of the matter to be voted on and, in the case of a proxy given to vote for the election of directors, shall list those persons who were nominees at the time of the notice of the vote for election of directors was given to the members. In any election of directors, any proxy which is marked by a member "withhold" or otherwise marked in a manner indicating that the authority to vote for the election of directors is withheld shall not be voted either for or against the election of a director.

If membership voting by proxy is allowed, proxies shall afford an opportunity for the members to specify a choice between approval and disapproval for each matter or group of related matters intended, at the time the proxy is distributed, to be acted upon at the meeting for which the proxy is solicited. The proxy shall also provide that when the person solicited specifies a choice with respect to any such matter, the vote shall be cast in accordance therewith.

Section 9. Conduct of Meetings. Meetings of members shall be presided over by the Chairperson of the Board, or, of there is no Chairperson, by the President of the corporation or, in his or her absence, by the Vice President of the corporation or, in the absence of all these persons, by a Chairperson chosen by a majority of the voting members, present in person or by proxy. The Secretary of the corporation shall act as Secretary of all meetings of members, provided that, in his or her absence, the presiding officer shall appoint another person to act as Secretary of the Meeting.

Meetings shall be governed by the rules of procedures, as such rules may be revised from time to time, insofar as such rules are not inconsistent with or in any conflict with these Bylaws, with the Articles of Incorporation of this corporation, or with any provision of law.

Section 10. Action By Written Ballot Without A Meeting. Any action which may be taken at any regular or special meeting of members may be taken without a meeting if the corporation distributes a written ballot to each member entitled to vote on the matter. The ballot shall set forth the proposed action, provide an opportunity to specify approval or disapproval of each proposal, provide that where the person solicited specifies a choice with respect to any such proposal the vote shall be cast in accordance therewith, and provide a reasonable time within which to return the ballot to the corporation. Ballots shall be mailed or delivered in the manner required for giving notice of meetings specified in Section 4 (b) of this Article.

All written ballots shall also indicate the number of responses needed to meet the quorum requirement and, except for ballots soliciting votes for the election of directors, shall state the percentage of approvals necessary to pass the measure submitted. The ballots must specify the time by which they must be received by the corporation in order to be counted.

Approval of action by written ballot shall be valid only when the number of votes cast by ballot within the time period specified equals or exceeds the quorum required to be present at a meeting authorizing the action, and the number of approvals equals or exceed the number of votes cast was the same number of votes cast by ballot.

Directors may be elected by written ballot. Such ballots for the election of directors shall list the persons nominated at the time the ballots are mailed or delivered. If any such ballots are marked "withhold" or otherwise marked in a manner indicating that the authority to vote for the election of directors is withheld, they shall not be counted as votes either for or against the election of a director.

A written ballot may not be revoked after its receipt by the corporation or its deposit in the mail, whichever occurs first.

Section 11. Reasonable Nomination and Election Procedures. This corporation shall make available to all members reasonable nomination and election procedure with respect to the election of directors by members. Such procedures shall be reasonable given the nature, size and operations of the corporation, and shall include:

(a). A reasonable means of nominating persons for election as directors.

(b). A reasonable opportunity for a nominee to communicate to the members the nominee's qualifications and the reasons for the nominees candidacy.

(c). A reasonable opportunity for all nominees to solicit votes.

(d). A reasonable opportunity for all members so choose among the nominees.

Upon the written request by any nominee for election to the Board and the payment with such request of the reasonable costs of mailing (including postage), the corporation shall, within ten (10) business days after such request (provided payment has been made) mail to all members or such portion of them that the nominee may reasonably specify, any material which the nominee shall furnish and which is reasonably related to the election, unless the corporation within five (5) business days after the request allows the nominee, at the corporation's option, the right to do either of the following:

1. Inspect and copy the record of all members' names, addresses and voting rights, at reasonable times, upon five (5) business days' prior written demand upon the corporation which demand shall state the purpose for which the inspection rights are requested; or

2. Obtain from the Secretary, upon written demand and payment of a reasonable charge, a list of the names, addresses and voting rights of those members entitled to vote for the election of directors, as of the most recent record date for which it has been compiled or as of any date specified by the nominee subsequent to the date of demand.

The demand shall state the purpose for which the list is requested and the membership list shall be made available on or before the later of ten (10) business days after the demand is received or after the date specified therein as the date as of which the list is to be compiled.

If the corporation distributes any written election material soliciting votes for any nominee for director at the corporation's expense, it shall make available, at the corporation's expense, to each other nominee, in or with the same material, the same amount of space that is provided any other nominee, with equal prominence, to be used by the nominee for a purpose reasonably related to the election.

Generally, any person who is qualified to be elected to the Board of Directors shall be nominated at the annual meeting of members held for the purpose of electing directors by any member present at the meeting in person or by proxy. However, if the corporation has five hundred (500) or more members, any of the additional nomination procedures specified in subsections (a) and (b) of Section 5221 of the California Nonprofit Public Benefit Corporation Law may be used to nominate persons for election to the Board of Directors.

Section 12. Action by Unanimous Written Consent Without Meeting.. Except as otherwise provided in these Bylaws, any action required or permitted to be taken by the members may be taken without a meeting, if all members shall individually or collectively consent in writing to the action. The written consent or consents shall be filed with the minutes of the proceedings of the members. The action by written consent shall have the same force and effect as the unanimous vote of the members.

Section 13. Record Date for Meetings. The record date for purposes of determining the members entitled to notice, voting rights, written ballot rights, or any other right with respect to a meeting of members or any other lawful membership action, shall be fixed pursuant to Section 5611 of the California Non-profit Public Benefit Corporation Law.

WRITTEN CONSENT OF DIRECTORS
ADOPTING BYLAWS

We, the undersigned, are all of the persons named as the initial directors in the Articles of Incorporation of Children of Uncle Sam Foundation, a California nonprofit corporation, and, pursuant to the authority granted to the directors by these Bylaws to take action by unanimous written consent without a meeting, consent to, and hereby do, adopt the foregoing Bylaws, consisting of _____ pages, as the Bylaws of this corporation.

Dated:_____

_____
Director

_____
Director

_____
Director

CERTIFICATE

This is to certify that the foregoing is a true and correct copy of the Bylaws of the corporation named in the title thereto and that such Bylaws were duly adopted by the Board of Directors of said corporation

Dated:_____

_____
Secretary

Corporate Seal

An Easy Guide On How to Establish Your First Residential Care Facility

EXHIBIT TWO: PROGRAM DESIGN

(SAMPLE ONLY)

ANGELCARE HOME

A RESIDENTIAL CARE FACILITY FOR ADULTS

A Sample Program Design

By: **HealthCare Training and Staffing Services**
3400 Inland Empire Boulevard, Suite 101
Ontario, Ca. 91764
(909) 484-1987

This program design is produced by HealthCare Training and Staffing Services, Incorporated. It is designed to provide factual and reliable information in an opinionated form. It is developed with the understanding that the publisher, editors, contributors and staff of this publication cannot be held responsible for any error (s) and omissions, nor any agency's interpretation, applications and changes of regulations described herein. Let it be expressly known that the author and staff of this publication are not rendering any professional, legal or technical advice or service. It is the responsibility of the clients whom the program design is awarded to keep themselves abreast of the latest rules and regulations in reference to the subject matter covered during the consultation session. The information presented herein is a collection of resources acquired from Title 22, Title 17 Regulation and other resources that are publicly available. This program design is exclusively made for, and doing business as Angelcare Home. No part of this publication/program design may be reproduced, copied, modified or transmitted in any form for any purpose and by any means, without the express written consent of HealthCare Training and Staffing Services, Incorporated.

All rights reserved, June 7, 2001 Ontario, California. USA

Table of Contents

Introduction 235
Mission Statement 236
The Uniqueness of the home: 236
THE COMPANY SUMMARY 236
Personnel Plan 238
Sample Personnel Schedule: 238
SERVICES OFFERED: 241
NURSING AND SOCIAL WORK 243
Activities: 245
Nutrition: 245
Transportation 246
PHYSICAL LAYOUT : Accessibility 247
Medical Equipment and Supplies 247
Physical Therapy 248
Exercise 248
Massage/ YOGA / Music Therapy 248
Music Therapy 248
Isolation and Illness 249
GROUP ACTIVITIES / TABLE TOP / RECREATION / ADAPTIVE SPORTS COGNITIVE TRAINING: 249
Consumers 251
ADMISSION CRITERIA 253
Schedule of Development : Time Line 255
Start Up Cost (Projections) 255
CONSUMER TRAINING TOPICS: 256
HEALTH CONDITIONS: Restricted Health Conditions: 264
Universal Precaution 265
RESTRICTED HEALTH CARE PLAN 270
Policies and Procedures 317
PLANNED ACTIVITIES OF COMMUNITY RESOURCES: 324
DISCHARGE/REMOVAL 325
CLOTHING: INITIAL CLOTHING: 326

PROCEDURES FOR SAFEGUARDING CLOTHING AND
PERSONAL PROPERTY: 327
RELIGIOUS SERVICES: 327
INTERNAL COMMUNICATION RECORD: 327

AngelCare HOME

A Residential Care Facility for Adults

Introduction

AngelCare Home, Residential Care Facility for Adults, *a level 4 residential care facility will be the county's best alternative to residential care setting for adults between the ages of 18 to over 59 years of age.*

AngelCare Home, Residential Care Facility for Adults is a comprehensive non-medical residential care designed specifically to serve the needs of adults with physical, social and/or developmental disability who need supervision and assistance on a 24 hour basis. It is a home developed to assist families and their loved ones in their temporary care and supervision as an alternative to an institutional setting such as a nursing home. The home is focused on improving the quality of health care services geared towards safety, health, social and other supportive services in a protective, friendly and non-institutional setting.

AngelCare Home, Residential Care Facility for Adults provides personalized care services including nursing, rehabilitation, activities, counseling, exercise, socialization, nutritious meals and snacks, and arrangements for transportation to and from the school or day program and other places of interest to the consumers.

The home is established as a result of an overwhelming demand for a unique type of a residential care setting that will provide personal care, vocational and habilitation training and mentorship, behavioral modification and therapy all under one service objective. The individualized program plan shall take into consideration the specific consumer needs and services, their functional ability, their challenges, their behaviors and their ability to retain and respond to given task.

Mission Statement

1. To provide the community with the best social, recreational, habilitative, behavioral, therapeutic activities and community integration program in a residential setting focused specifically on the disabled adult population.

2. To establish an excellent setting for residential care where individuals with physical, behavioral, developmental, social and medical challenges achieve their utmost potentials in life.

The Uniqueness of the home:

AngelCare Home, Residential Care Facility for Adults offers a unique adult residential care 24 hour non-medical setting focused on the individualized consumer's needs and services, disabilities, potentials, learning curve, behaviors and most of all to enhance the consumers' social and recreational skills. **AngelCare Home, Residential Care Facility for Adults** offers a wide variety of activities, behavior modification components, therapy, and mentorship.

THE COMPANY SUMMARY

AngelCare Home, Incorporated is a company that will establish a residential care facility in the Sample City and shall call it **AngelCare Home, a 6-Bed Residential Care Facility for Adults.** It shall rise above the standards of an average residential care setting as it will introduce a unique approach to activities, therapy, community integration, and socialization. This will be totally different and non-conventional in approach compared to the average residential care home in a sense that the program design is focused mainly on the individual client's needs which is ever changing and not based as a group setting.

The business address of the company shall be located at 12345 Same Street, Sample City, Ca. 91234. Contact person is Sample Joe, Administrator. The initial board of directors are as follows:

An Easy Guide On How to Establish Your First Residential Care Facility

Mr. John Sample, President
Mrs. Yunmi Sample, Vice President
Ms. Jason Sample, Secretary-Treasurer

AngelCare Home, Residential Care Facility for Adults shall be managed and administered by Ms. Yuri Sample, Facility Administrator.

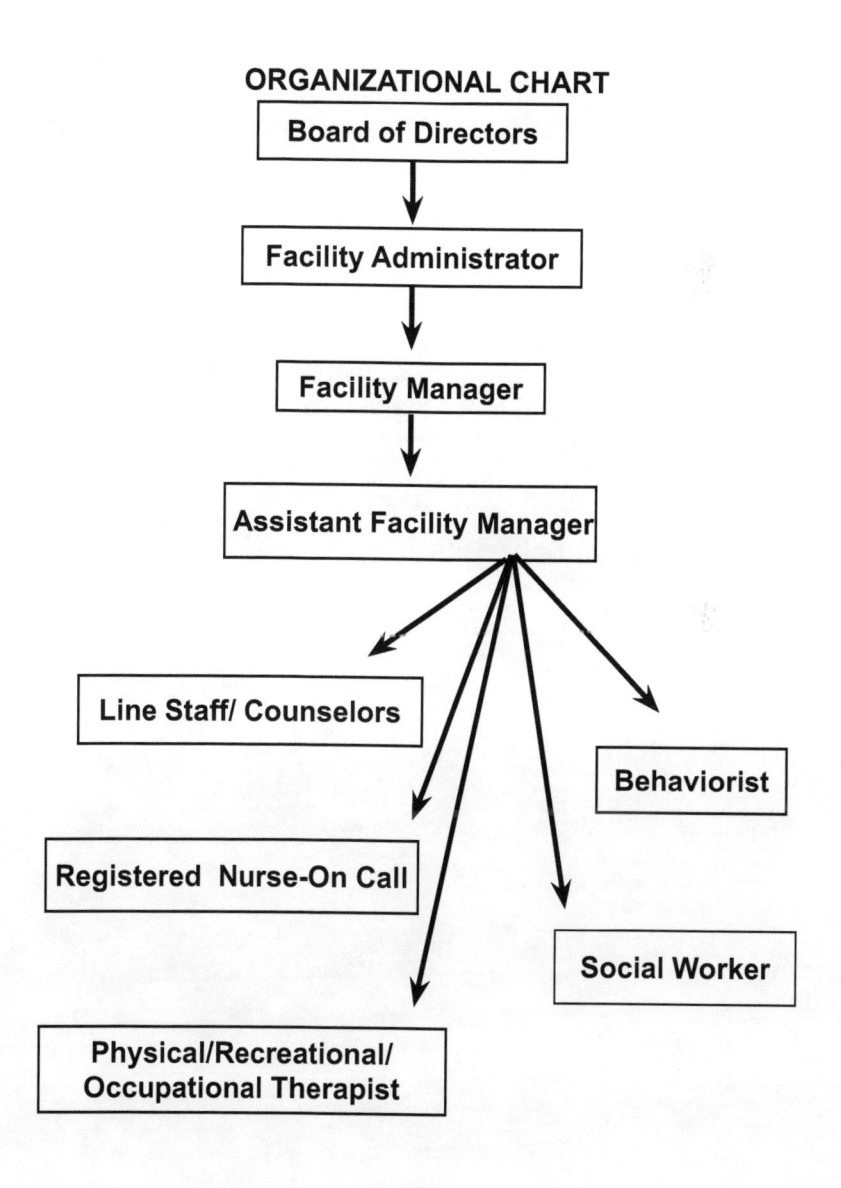

ORGANIZATIONAL CHART

Board of Directors
↓
Facility Administrator
↓
Facility Manager
↓
Assistant Facility Manager
↓
- Line Staff/ Counselors
- Behaviorist
- Registered Nurse-On Call
- Social Worker
- Physical/Recreational/ Occupational Therapist

Personnel Plan

The initial set of personnel shall consist of Facility Administrator, Facility Manager who shall hire initial two direct care staff and support staff during the first three weeks of operation to accommodate the first group of residents. As the population of consumers increases, so is the number of staff to increase in proportion to the population of consumers placed in the home.

The staffing ratio is 1 staff to 3 consumers. However, when the company starts accepting consumers who have behavior issues as well as those with considerable amount of community involvement and social recreation, the number of staff to consumer ratio shall be increased considerably in proportion to the dictates of the program statement which must meet the needs of the consumers accordingly. Our standard staffing ratio considering our consumer/client population will be at 1:3 on a daily basis. There may be clients with behaviors and in such case when the demand for closer supervision and monitoring, the staffing ratio in that case, will be increased to 1:1.

Sample Personnel Schedule:

AngelCare Home, Residential Care Facility for Adults

Note: Staff No. represents the staff ID No. (Sample Staff 0.1)

An Easy Guide On How to Establish Your First Residential Care Facility

WK End	Day	Mon 7:00a 2:00p	Tue 7:00a 2:00p	Wed 7:00a 2:00p	Thu 7:00a 2:00p	Fri 7:00a 2:00p
	1	Staff 0.1	Staff 0.1	Staff 0.1	Staff 0.12	Staff 0.12
	2	Staff 0.12	Staff 0.12	Staff 0.12	Staff 0.12	Staff 0.12
	3	Staff 0.13	Staff 0.13	Staff 4	Staff 4	Staff 4
	4	Staff 4	Staff 0.13	Staff 4	Staff 0.12	Staff 0.12
	5	Staff 5	Staff 0.13	Staff 4	Staff 0.12	Staff 0.12
6		Staff 6	Staff 0.13	Staff 4	Staff 0.12	Staff 0.12
7		Staff 6	Staff 0.13	Staff 4	Staff 0.12	Staff 0.12
	8	Staff 8	Staff 8	Staff 7	Staff 8	Staff 8
	9	Staff 9	Staff 9	Staff 8	Staff 9	Staff 9
	10	Staff 10	Staff 10	Staff 9	Staff 10	Staff 10
	11	Staff 0.13	Staff 0.13	Staff 10	Staff 0.12	Staff 0.12
	12	Staff 10	Staff 10	Staff 9	Staff 10	Staff 10
13		Staff 7	Staff 7	Staff 4	Staff 7	Staff 7
14		Staff 7	Staff 7	Staff 4	Staff 7	Staff 7
	15	Staff 0.1	Staff 0.1	Staff 0.1	Staff 0.12	Staff 0.12

	16	Staff 0.12	Staff 0.12	Staff 0.12	Staff 0.12	Staff 0.12
	17	Staff 0.13	Staff 0.13	Staff 4	Staff 4	Staff 4
	18	Staff 0.13	Staff 4	Staff 0.12	Staff 0.12	Staff 0.13
	19	Staff 0.13	Staff 4	Staff 0.12	Staff 0.12	Staff 0.13
20		Staff 0.13	Staff 4	Staff 0.12	Staff 0.12	Staff 0.13
21		Staff 0.12	Staff 0.12	Staff 0.12	Staff 0.12	Staff 0.12
	22	Staff 0.13	Staff 0.13	Staff 4	Staff 4	Staff 4
	23	Staff 0.13	Staff 4	Staff 0.12	Staff 0.12	Staff 0.13
	24	Staff 0.13	Staff 4	Staff 0.12	Staff 0.12	Staff 0.13
	25	Staff 0.13	Staff 4	Staff 0.12	Staff 0.12	Staff 0.13
	26	Staff 0.12	Staff 0.12	Staff 0.12	Staff 0.12	Staff 0.12
27		Staff 4	Staff 0.13	Staff 4	Staff 0.12	Staff 0.12
28		Staff 5	Staff 0.13	Staff 4	Staff 0.12	Staff 0.12
	29	Staff 6	Staff 0.13	Staff 4	Staff 0.12	Staff 0.12
	30	Staff 6	Staff 0.13	Staff 4	Staff 0.12	Staff 0.12

SERVICES OFFERED:

AngelCare Home, Residential Care Facility for Adults shall offer the highest quality in residential care programming activities to be able to accommodate six residents in a beautiful three bedroom home setting. The program believes in the principle... " that every resident must be treated with dignity and respect at all times". Regardless of the consumers' needs whether it be behavioral, emotional or psychological, an individualized personal plan shall be developed in a personalized manner to accommodate the residents' needs and to keep them active within the home and in a broad sense, for the residents to maintain a lifestyle of normalcy, integration and independence.

AngelCare Home, Residential Care Facility for Adults shall offer the following component services with emphasis on the clients' choice, rights and self-advocacy :

1. **Creative Learning:** Focused primarily on providing the consumers with creative and functional-educational activities, to offer a learning and nurturing environment to develop their much needed skills and provide an all natural, unrestricted environment of free choice for personal development and growth through learning. In order to achieve this, the home shall exert its best effort and resources in maximizing the utilization of community resources, funding and support from other entities, public agencies as well as private entities.

2. **Independent Living:** Provide much needed independent living skills that the consumers/clients shall learn as part of their goal to attain a lifestyle of self-reliance and personal growth. The facility objective is focused on functional skills and personal needs of the consumers/clients. The home will provide an environment of learning for adaptation and habilitation where provision for supervised training on the use of home equipments, cooking utensils etc.. is applied. The goal is to familiarize the consumers on the life of self-reliance and independence by learning to cook, prepare their own meal, housekeeping and home maintenance.

3. **Personal Development:** In order to develop personal, social, recreational, tactile and other related skills, the home will promote the individualized development of personal self-care, meal preparation, feeding, occupational and recreational skills by providing age appropriate equipment, tools of learning and resources needed to enhance the individuals personal capacity. The consumers will be treated to a monthly trip to special places of interest such as museums, parks, camping trips, trips to the casino and other interesting places that consumers prefer in order to enhance their social and recreational skills.

4. **Community Integration.** To promote consumer's self-reliance and confidence the home will provide supervised training staff to assists the consumers in community participation and to enhance their personal experiences within the community by facilitating positive interaction with others, within the community and of course their own home environment or community. The home shall provide training, assistance and support in various areas of community integration. Part of the consumer's learning expectations include safety at home and in public, parenting skills, mobility training and assistance in accessing community resources.

5. **Job Training and Supervision.** The home shall provide learning in career counseling, planning and mentoring through staff supervision. The home shall provide learning skills and tools needed in the advancement of the consumer's lifestyle through computer learning, resume writing and personal correspondence.

6. **Physical, recreational, occupational and emotional therapy.** The home shall provide the consumers with activities that will enhance their physical, recreational and emotional needs such as morning exercises, walks to the parks, aromatherapy, interactive-music, computer familiarization, Friday and Saturday dance nights and Karaoke nights, etc... The consumers will be taken to a public areas, dance halls, parks, city parks and recreation etc.. where they will participate in community participation where they will go out into the community to do volunteer clean ups of churches, beaches, parks and recreation to show their support to the community.

7. **Behavior modification.** In order to keep the consumers active in the home and in the community, consumers who may have behavior or emotional issues will be provided with a 1:1 or an average of 3:1 staff to consumer ratio in the event that they become non-conforming. An in-house behaviorist will be available to draw up a program plan to address their individual behavior which will be executed by a staff familiar with the consumer in particular.

8. **Transition planning:** Proving the consumer(s) with a learning program to help them learn the basics of Independent living such as lessons in cooking, gardening, safety, self-reliance in case of an emergency, food and material purchasing, budgeting, money management, housekeeping, job search and interviewing, etc...

9. **Transportation:** The program shall include availability of transportation through staff transport, a non-mobile/mobile van/bus to transport the consumers to and from their homes and other locations relative to their needs and services.

NURSING AND SOCIAL WORK

AngelCare Home, Residential Care Facility for Adults will provide a variety of non-medical, and social service needs. The home will be licensed in accordance with Title 22 and Title 17 Regulation. The home will be vendorized and licensed by the Department of Health Services, Dept. of Social Services, Community care Licensing and Dept of Developmental Services, Inland Regional Center, Health Care Licensing and other Government Agencies. Medical and Mental / Behavioral issues are monitored by a registered nurse and a social worker on staff. Both should be knowledgeable and experienced in meeting the psychological and social needs of the residents. The Registered Nurse will be retained as a regular staff present at the home while the residents are present. Staff is expected to provide medication monitoring and reminders. The staff is likewise trained on a regular basis to monitor the following client needs:

Medication administration and management.
Blood pressure/weight
Bladder training and/or continence
Nutrition instruction and special diet
Specific nursing procedures
Personal care services
Bathing, Hair care
Assistance with meals
Arrange for speech, physical, recreational and behavior therapy orcounseling

There shall be a social worker on staff who will provide a therapeutic counseling, information, referral services, caregiver support groups, Individual, group, and/or family counseling,

Types of nursing services available:

1. Medication administration and management.
2. Blood pressure/weight
3. Bladder training and/or continence
4. Nutrition instruction and special diet
5. Stool monitoring

Personal care services

1. Bathing
2. Hair care
3. Assistance with meals
4. Assistance in Activities of Daily Living

Other Services:

1. Speech therapy
2. Recreation therapy
3. Physical therapy
4. Social work services
5. Information and referral
6. Individual, group, and/or family counseling
7. Transportation to The Home and transportationto other places for appointments, shopping, etc...
8. Medical assessment

9. Medical Treatment
10. Onsite podiatry care
11. Art therapy
12. Music therapy
13. Reality therapy
14. Exercises
15. Assistance dressing/grooming/using the toilet

Activities:

One of the benefits of participating in the Home is for the consumers to receive excellent personalized services and activities that is significant to their well being. The program of activities offered will be diverse, focusing on mental and physical stimulation, the strengths and interests of the residents.

There will be a designated lead staff who will implement activity designs that are suited to meet the capabilities and potentials of each and every individual resident at the Home that is diverse, stimulating, interactive and enjoyable. The residents are encouraged to take part in activities on a regular basis. There will be opportunities for individual or small group activities.

Pottery making, gardening, arts and crafts, games, dancing, exercises, computer-Internet, participate in a play or stage presentation etc....

Nutrition:

Proper nutrition plays an important role in preserving the health of our residents. The Home shall provide a minimum of three meals and two snacks a day. The dining area will be conducive to a relaxing meal, with tables placed to encourage socialization. The dining area will be maintained in clean and orderly, attractive, well-lit, and inviting at all times.

Special diets are often necessary for residents. Those meals, as well as the standard meals, will also be appetizing, tasty and attractively served as well as a regular meal. The Home shall also provide meals that are calorie controlled, kosher, vegetarian or meet the special requirements of diabetics, provide supplemental feedings or pureed foods provided when necessary.

Over-all, the dining room area will be warm, congenial atmosphere and inviting at all times. During meals, there shall be at least one staff member for every six residents. Volunteers cannot be counted as part of this ratio.

Residents will be served with a well-balance diet consisting of the six basic food groups and prepared by an in-house cook or outsourced from a food preparer.

Sample meals: Menus will be available upon request which will be updated every month, one week in advance.

Transportation

AngelCare Home, Residential Care Facility for Adults, shall provide accessible transportation on a regular and timely manner. There shall be a designated van or bus to transport both ambulatory and non-ambulatory residents. **AngelCare Home,** shall also authorize the use its staff transportation to accommodate individual or group activities specifically those attending community based programming.

There shall be experienced and trained transporter and shall undergo regular safety training sponsored by **AngelCare Home,** or from any available training resources. The transportations will be maintained in safe and working condition where a transportation maintenance and mileage log will be retained. There shall be an available aide on the van who will assist the driver in loading and unloading of the residents.

There shall be safety equipment present and available at the van at all times. Prior to transporting all belt will be fastened to secure the safety of the residents and there will be a radio or cellular phone available for emergencies.

PHYSICAL LAYOUT : Accessibility

AngelCare Home, shall be accessible to disabled individuals, specialized equipment will be installed or structural modifications will be made to ensure such accessibility (e.g., ramps, grab bars, wide doorways and turning spaces for wheelchairs).

The Home shall consult with the local city planning department, the local Licensing District Office, or the State Department of Rehabilitation, Community Access/Rehabilitation Engineering Section. (Please see site sketch)

- Equipment and Supplies

Medical Equipment and Supplies

1. Airways
2. Emergency oxygen supply and equipment for administration
3. Examination light
4. First aid and emergency supplies
5. Flashlights
6. Medicine glasses, cups, or other small calibrated containers
7. Refrigerator with thermometer
8. Weight scale
9. Commode chairs, wheelchairs, walkers, canes, crutches
10. Soap for bathing
11. Sphygmomanometer
12. Sterile dressing
13. Stethoscope
14. Syringes and needles
15. Supplies to perform urine and acetone testing
16. Thermometers
17. Tongue depressors
18. Current drug reference listing indications for use, dosage, range, and side effects
19. Locked cabinet for storage of medications

Physical Therapy

1. Parallel bars (Portable/Collapsible)
2. Overhead pulley and weights
3. Set of training stairs
4. Treatment table
5. Availability of wheelchairs, walkers, canes, crutches, and other ambulatory aids
6. Other equipment and supplies as needed for specific therapy modalities

Exercise

The Home will be equipped with the free weights, dumb bells, exercise equipments that are appropriate to the needs of our consumers.

Occupational Therapy:

1. Equipment and supplies for evaluation and training of fine motor skills and sensory integration
2. Supplies for adaptive equipment for reeducation in activities of daily living
3. Equipment and supplies for creative skills such as leatherwork, needlework, ceramics, woodworking, painting, and graphic arts.

Massage/ YOGA / Music Therapy

Residents who have spasticity and other muscle and joint issues will benefit from a therapeutic massage where a trained staff will provide muscle toning and water therapy. The Home will be equipped with a folding portable massage table and softened floor mats where residents will be able to lay down and roll over on a therapeutic ball; soak their feet in a vibrating wash basin while they listen to a soft classical music to soothe their aching pains.

Music Therapy

1 Stereo/CD Player

2. Soft lights and inviting colorful room
3. Big pillows
4. Soft plastic floors
5. Natural sound tapes and audio visuals
6. Colorful soft tone pictures and posters.

Isolation and Illness

AngelCare Home shall be equipped with a stethoscope, thermometer, blood sugar tester, a small refrigerator to keep medications, a hospital type bed, an oxygen tank, and other non-medical, non-emergency equipment to support residents with medical related needs.

There will be a designated nurse on site who will do the diagnosis and evaluation, and there will also be a physician who is on call and available when ever the need for consultation and evaluation is needed.

GROUP ACTIVITIES / TABLE TOP / RECREATION / ADAPTIVE SPORTS COGNITIVE TRAINING:

VOCATIONAL SKILLS DEVELOPMENT WHICH INCLUDES ACADEMICS, BASIC LETTER WRITING & NAME IDENTIFICATION, AND CALENDAR RECOGNITION.

SKILL: SENSORY MOTOR STIMULATION, BUILDING SOCIAL AND COMMUNICATION SKILLS. LEARNING ABOUT TEXTURES, SMELLS, COLORS, SAFETY, ETC., INFORMALLY LEARN TO PUT THINGS ON/IN TARGET, UTILIZE VARIETY OF ITEMS TO CREATE PROJECTS.

TABLE TOP GAMES: INTRO TO VARIOUS GAMES; INFORMALLY TEACH HOW TO TAKE TURNS, HOW TO MOVE OBJECTS, GAME PIECES AND COOPERATIVE, PLAY; AND COMMUNICATION SKILLS.

COOKING CLASS: INFORMAL TRAINING ON HOW TO READ A RECIPE, MEASURE INGREDIENTS, POUR, STIR AND MIX. PREPARATION FOR SNACK AT SNACK TIME AS APPROPRIATE.

DOMESTIC SKILLS: INFORMAL/FORMAL TRAINING TO SET TABLE AND PREPARE FOR MEAL PER ISP OBJ.

FOOD ART: MAKING CRAFT OBJECTS FROM THINGS FOUND IN THE KITCHEN, MAKING FOOD (JELLO JIGGLERS, ETC.) THAT CAN BE EATEN FOR SNACK ON FRIDAY, MAKING SENSORY PLAYDOUGH THAT HAS SMELL/TACTILE STIMULATION.

ART/PAINT PROJECT: MAKE A PAINTING WITH ASSORTED COLORS OF WTERCOLORS; FINGERPAINTS, WASHABLE PAINTS ON THE ARTBOARD PAPER USING FINGERS/BRUSHES/ROLLERS, ETC.

ART: INFORMAL TEACHING, CREATING CRAFT PROJECTS USING VARIETY OF ITEMS, PAPER, CHALK, MAATERIALS, JEWELRY, FEATHERS, ETC.

TABLE TOP ART: INFORMAL TRAINING ON HOW TO MOLD AND SHAPE CLAY CREATE DIFFERENT OBJECTS. COLOR & TEXTURE AWARENESS.

GARDENING SKILLS: INFORMAL TEACHING ON HOW TO WATER THE YARD & PLANTS.

HOW TO CULTIVATE SOIL & PLANT SEEDS & PLANT CARE.

MUSICAL BAND: INFORMAL TARINING ON HOW TO HOLD AND MAKE SOUNDS WITH VARIOUS MUSICAL INRUMENTS, OFFERING OPPORTUNITY FOR CHOICES.

MUSIC EXERCISE: SENSORY MOTOR STIMULATION, INTRODUCTION TO VARIOUS EXERCISE TECHNIQUES, ROM TRAINING TO DIFFERENT SOUNDS AND RYTHMS OF MUSIC, FOLLOWING PHYSICAL THERAPISTS RECOMMENDATION FOR INDIVIDUAL. ROM TO MUSIC VIDEO.

MOBILITY TRAINING: TO DEVELOP ECH CLIENTS INDEPENDENCE TO BE MOBILE WITHIN THEIR ENVIRONMENT, BOTH IN THE COMMUNITY AND AT HOME.

ADAPTIVE SPORTS: INFORMAL TRAINING ON HOW TO THROW/ROLL/CATCH/PASS A BALL OR OTHER OBJECT, BASKETBALL, BOWLING, VELCRO DARTS, ETC.

COMMUNITY OUTING: INFORMALLY WORK ON APPROPRIATE SOCIAL BEHAVIOR, COMMUNICATION SKILLS AND PURCHASING SKILLS.

COMMUNITY AWARENESS: TRAINING IN LOCATION IDENTIFICATION, OBJECT IDENTIFICATION (FLOWER, TREE, COLOR, CAR, NEIGHBORS, ETC.) COLLECT ITEMS SUCH AS LEAVES, FLOWERS, ACORNS, ETC FOR ART/CRAFT PROJECT FOR THURSDAY OR FRIDAY. (NATURE WALKS, PICNICS).

COMMUNICATION SKILL: INFORMAL/FORMAL TRAINING COORDINATED THROUGHOUT THA DAY WITHIN ALL ACTIVITIES, TO DEVELOP RECEPTIVE AND EXPRESSIVE COMMUNICATION.

DISCUSSION OF CURRENT EVENTS: INFORMAL TRAINING TO DEVELOP SOCIAL SKILLS, AWARENESS OF DAILY EVENTS IN THEIR PERSONAL LIVES.

REST & RELAXATION PERIOD:
CLIENTS RELAX AND LISTEN TO MUSIC ON RADIO OR TAPES & SOCIAIZE WITH PEERS.

Story Time

BOOKS ON TAPE, BOOKS READ ALOUD, CORRESPONDING PUPPETRY SKILL: COMMUNICATION, CORRELATION OF COLOR TO PICTURE OF COLOR, SENSORU TOUCH BOOKS TO FEELING, ETC.

Consumers

AngelCare Home consumers shall comprise of individuals with developmental disability who are primarily adults and seniors from the Regional Center who may have minor medical issues, those with dual diagnosis and possibly having behavior issues such as mild psychotic and institution like pattern of behavior that is observed to be on an on-going basis. For the safety and well-being of all our resident consumers, the home will be formulating behavior modification plans for consumers who seem to be non-compliant and aggressive in nature and to possibly allocate a behavior area to be able to address their personal issues.

Another focal point of reference shall be the variety of services we will provide to our consumers, the quality of our services which follows the highest standard of care and supervision, our consistency in our staffing ratio to consumers which is an average of 1:3 to maintain high quality standard as well as continuous training of our staff and most of all our focus on safety and cleanliness at the home to make it conducive for interaction, learning and a good working environment for our consumers as well as our staff.

The key element in our home is our excellent relationship between staff and the consumers, with Regional Center Social Workers.

The following factors are our asset:

1. Quality of care and supervision which upholds the highest standards
2. Safety and cleanliness.
3. Staffing based on the program offered which requires courtesy, respect, freedom from abuse and neglect, experience and education maintained by the staff in general.
4. Continuous staff training and in-services / certification on medication monitoring, risk and safety management and proper client care and supervision.
5. Program variety, practical application and consistency.
6. Consistency in programming and follow-up on consumer's progress and development.
7. How the consumers will be able to learn and enjoy their activities that address their needs and services.

It is however of utmost importance for the consumers to be able to enjoy the activities we offer at home and their ability to conform with our house rules and policies.

ADMISSION CRITERIA

1. Must have a Developmental Disability. The disabilities may include: a diagnosis of mild to profound mental retardation, autism, cerebral palsy and epilepsy. Individuals may have a dual diagnosis with on-going behavior problems and/or may have mild severe physical challenges. Physical challenges may include: the use of wheelchairs, needing assistance with hygiene, transferring and other personal needs.

2. Must be at least eighteen (18) years of age up to 59 +

3. Should be referred by the Regional Center, Dept. of Aging and other Government Services Agencies.

4. Must possess the potential to benefit from program services determined by the intake application, case records and evaluation process.

5. Must be free of behavioral conditions which pose a hazard to the consumer, others and/or property.

6. May be willing to accept individuals with a history of on-going assaultive behavior and property damage.

7. Will accept individuals with health conditions which require incidental medical services, provided that the medical condition(s) are chronic and stable, temporary in nature and are expected to return to a condition normal for that individual is under the medical care of a licensed professional.

8. Must be able to conform with the regulation, the house rules and policies.

9. Will accept both ambulatory and non-ambulatory consumers.

10. Must be in the process of acquiring self-help skills.

11. Will provide feeding assistance to those consumers in need.

12. Will provide transfer assistance to consumers in wheelchairs. If a lift device is required, this must be provided by another entity.

13. Will accept consumers who wear adult briefs.

14. Will accept ensure that incontinent consumers are checked at regular intervals and are kept clean.

15. Will accept consumers who require scheduled toileting at regular intervals.

16. Will provide assistance to consumers who can benefit from scheduled toileting by assisting or reminding them to go to the bathroom at regular intervals.

17. Will accept consumers who require assistance in hygiene and self-care tasks.

18. Will provide all necessary assistance to consumers in need.

19. Will not accept individuals who require health services or have a prohibited health condition(s) including:
    1. Naso-gastric and naso-duodenal tubes.
    2. Staph infection or other serious infection.
    3. Active, communicable TB.
    4. Conditions which require 24 hour nursing care or oversight.
    5. Stage 3 or 4 decubitus ulcers.
    6. Any other condition or care requirements which would require the Association to be licensed as a health facility

An Easy Guide On How to Establish Your First Residential Care Facility

Schedule of Development : Time Line

2002 Apr May Jun Jul Aug Sep Oct Nov Dec Jan **2003**

1. Proposal Submission: ↔-------→
2. Program Design: ↔-↔
3. Program Submission: ←--------→
4. Finish Home Construction: ←----→
5. Program Review: ↔↔↔↔↔↔↔↔↔↔
6. Program Revision / approval: ↔↔↔↔↔
7. Facility Location/Development: ↔ ↔↔↔↔
8. Meet Title 22 and 17 Guidelines ↔↔↔↔↔
9. Fingerprinting ↔↔↔↔↔↔↔
10. Site visit/IRC-Licensing: ↔↔↔↔
11. Fire Marshall certification: ↔------------↔
12. Purchase of day program materials and equipment:
    ---↔↔↔↔↔↔----------------
13. Staff hiring and training ↔↔↔
14. Marketing
15. Initial Operation -----------↔↔
16. Consumers Start ↔↔↔↔↔↔

Start Up Cost (Projections)

The start up cost for **AngelCare Home** is approximately $67,000.00 to pay for our initial fixed and variable costs as well as to meet our expenses in developing our home site. We project based on conservative estimates that approximately $26,899.00 will be spend effectively for our expenses on the application process, office equipment and supplies, equipment and supplies.

During our initial operation, we will be utilizing our investors funds to register our company with the Secretary of State of California. After registration, we will be purchasing office equipment and supplies, facility equipment and tables, chairs and cabinets, educational materials to decorate our site. Most of the furniture will be purchased from an auction sale and shall be in very good condition which will be integrated with our facility design patterned after functional and practical purposes.

Start up cost:

Table 6.1 Start-Up Cost (See sample)

Financial Considerations

Revenues

a. Reimbursement for Services

    Medi-Cal:
    Private pay:
    Dept. of Aging
    Dept. of Rehab
    Other sources:

1. Grants (public and private)
2. Cash donations
3. In-kind contributions
4. Fund-raising events
5. Veteran's Administration
6. UMTA 16B2 grants for transportation
7. Adult Day Care Food Program

CONSUMER TRAINING TOPICS:

- Recreation/Leisure
- Travel Training
- Personal Care
- Health and Safety Awareness
- Medication Management
- Nutrition & Meal Preparation
- Self-Identity, Personal Adjustment, Communication, Civic Awareness & Responsibility
- Vocational Development

- Functional Academics
- Consumer Skills
- Behavior Management
- Other Supports As Needed

Training Techniques and Approaches

Training Techniques includes individual and group instruction, individual and group counseling, behavior modification, community instruction and classroom instruction.

LOCATION(S) OF CONSUMER TRAINING:

Group sessions will be conducted in a class environment and, when possible, in the appropriate community location. All training that consists of community resources such as shopping, banking, etc. will be conducted in the natural environment of the surrounding neighborhood.

A. **Recreation/Leisure:** Staff will instruct the consumers in choosing appropriate leisure time activities. Staff will emphasize the benefits of community-based recreation and leisure activities.

- Helps you unwind on weekends before a new week begins
- Opportunities to meet new people
- Exposure to different social situations and use of skills, such as communication skills, proper dress and appropriate grooming
- Exposure to different cultures
- Exercise through sports
- Learning about surroundings
- Increasing knowledge (Example: Museums, Lectures)

Consumers will also receive instructions on how to choose a recreational activity, including:

- Consumer interest
- Budget – What you can afford

- Availability
- Choose of recreational activities
- Different types of parties: Selecting an appropriate party for holidays, birthdays and different occasions, formal to informal, dinner to movies
- The different occasions
- The locations
- The type of entertainment
- Consumers will learn to use natural resources in making arrangements for recreation and leisure; such s, newspapers, phone books, etc.
- Planning a menu for appropriate number of people
- Invitations

Planning a Trip:

- Deciding where to go
- Amount of money needed
- Food arrangements
- Attractions or tours, cost, times

Making Reservations:

- Decide location and motel
- Stay in motel or with friends
- Calling ahead for cost and information

B. **Travel Training:** Consumers will receive training to ride public transportation for community integration activities. Training will include actual travel to/from the program to the following possible locations:

- Shopping Centers
- Recreational Events
- Restaurants
- Employment Sites

Training will be given on:

- Locating bus stops
- Selecting the proper bus

- Transferring buses
- Paying bus fares
- Debarking the bus
- Pedestrian laws
- Bus schedules

C. **Personal Self-Care & Hygiene:** Staff will assist consumers in presenting themselves to the public in an acceptable manner. Modern, age appropriate clothing, coupled with a clean body and attractive hair style will be the focus to establish self-esteem, as well as, presenting a well groomed image to the public. For those consumers who are in need of assistance with their self-care tasks, staff will provide all necessary supports.

The focus will be on the following areas:

- Discuss and role play how to recognize when a bath or shower is necessary
- Discuss and demonstrate how to maintain their own hair
- Discuss and demonstrate proper way to brush teeth and gums
- Discuss and play with female consumers how to take the proper care needed during her menstrual cycle
- Discuss and demonstrate how to present a neat appearance
- Discuss and demonstrate how to care for their shaving needs, including the use of various related appliances and toilet articles
- Discuss and demonstrate how to care for their clothes properly
- Discuss and demonstrate how to properly care for nails

D. **Health & Safety Awareness; Medication Management:** Consumers will learn, in a group as well as on an individual basis, Emergency Procedures:

- What to do in case of fire
- What to do in case of a disaster
- What to do in case of an accident
- What to do in case of illness

- How to use basic first aid techniques in treating minor injuries
- What to do if someone is having a seizure
- What to do if someone is choking
- When calling a police, what information do you need to tell them
- The identification and safe storage of poisons
- Keeping floors and walkway areas clear of hazardous objects
- How to obtain hard to reach items and how to lift heavy items
- Safe use of electrical outlets and appliances
- How to operate a flashlight and understand its value as an emergency appliance
- Use of fire extinguisher
- Discussion of awareness of medications taken, their need, and dosages
- Teach proper use of over-the-counter drugs and medicines not requiring a prescription
- Emergency phone numbers: Police, Fire, Doctor, Pharmacy, Etc.
- Discussion of services provided by medical care facilities

Disaster and Fire Drills will be conducted at random every month. Staff will time the consumers and note in a Disaster/Fire Log the time and any concerns. The staff will also discuss the drill with the consumers. Both the consumers and staff will discuss any concerns they may have.

E. **Nutrition & Meal Preparation:** Staff will instruct consumers on Nutrition & Basic Cooking & Meal Preparation Tasks in small group settings and on an individual basis. Staff will train consumers to prepare their morning snacks, as well as, provide training in lunch preparation skills. (Example: Use of microwave, cutting sandwiches, pouring beverages). Training will also be provided in preparing simple food items.

The consumers will learn & shall also demonstrate the use of:

- Pots & pans for cooking purposes
- Safe use of knife

- Measurements
- Kitchen techniques such as chopping, paring, grating, baking, broiling, boiling, frying
- The proper food storage
- Safe use of stove & oven
- Proper & safe use of kitchen appliances (Example: garbage disposal, toaster, coffee pot, electric mixer, microwave oven)

F. Self-Advocacy, Self-Identity, Personal Adjustment, Interpersonal Relations & Communication: The Home will focus on each individual's needs in learning Self-Advocacy Skills. The focus will be, but not limited to, the following areas:

- Knowing their rights
- Learning to say no
- Obtaining & requesting assistance
- Learning to express their own view point
- Speaking out in an appropriate manner
- Making informed choices

Self-Identity, Personal Adjustment, Interpersonal Relations & Communication Skills include:

- Use of personal identification
- Discussion of wishes 7 desires
- Development of goals
- Discussion & demonstration of getting along with others
- Discussion of issue of privacy, respecting others & appropriate social behavior
- Discussion & demonstration of basic communication skills

G. **Consumer Skills:** Consumer will learn shopping / consumer skills in the natural environment. Staff will train consumers in the following areas:

- To buy simple items
- To request assistance from salesperson when needed
- To shop for bargains
- To verbalize information about types of stores

- To exchange items
- To exhibit appropriate behavior in stores
- To locate products in different areas of stores
- To purchase items appropriate to need
- To purchase food in a restaurant or take-out shop
- To purchase items from vending machines & other coin-operated machines

H. **Functional Academics**: Staff will instruct consumers in Functional Academic Skills in small group settings and on an individual basis. Functional Academic Skills Training will include: Functional Reading

- Functional Writing
- Functional Academics
- Functional Consumer Skills

Training will be provided in the natural environment and will include:

- Identification of important personal data
- Responding appropriately to written information on watches, clocks & other dials & gauges
- Responding appropriately to written information found on safety signs, size labels, price tags & other signs & labels
- Locating needed information from simple charts, diagrams, maps & menus
- Carrying out simple directions written on packages, machinery, equipment & items that are assembled
- Responding appropriately to key words found on employment forms & other simple blanks & forms
- Identifying help wanted ads, printed advertisements, correspondence & other written materials & will seek the assistance of a responsible person to decode written & printed material that he/she is unable to read
- Carrying out transactions involving money (Example: pay telephone, bus fare, vending machines)
- Identifying situations involving time (Example: day of week, month of the year, seasons, major holidays, arriving on time to scheduled activities & events)

I. **Vocational Development:** Consumers will learn in a group setting as on an individual basis Work Adjustment Skills required for job placement. These skills will include the following areas:

- Seek help when needed
- To remain in work area until all work is completed
- Report to work on time
- Following instructions
- Identifying mistakes
- Correcting mistakes
- Completes work with supervisor independently
- Refraining from unnecessary social communication on job
- Accepting supervision
- Accepting criticism
- Following supervisor's suggestions
- Cooperating with co-workers
- Reporting emergencies
- Following correct time schedule for breaks & lunch
- Calls employer when unable to get to work
- Verbalizes correct information about employee's role
- Verbalizes correct information about employee/supervisor relationship
- Identifies own skills
- Identifies skills needed for job area of interest
- Identifies need for additional training
- Makes voluntary effort to acquire additional training
- Identifies possible employment resources
- Demonstrates correct interviewing procedure

In addition to Work Adjustment Training, consumers will have opportunities to develop their vocational skills through center based packaging & assembly type work, enclave placement in community settings & volunteer placements. Examples of employment environment to be pursued for job experience are the following:

1. Eating & Drinking Establishments: Fast food, Cafeterias, Restaurants
2. Food Stores: Grocery, Bakeries

3. Miscellaneous Retail: Drug, Used Merchandise, Shopping Stores
4. Hospitality: Hotels, Motels
5. Amusement & Recreation Services: Dance Studios, Schools, Health/Recreational Clubs
6. Health Services: Medical Clinics & Offices, Hospitals, Nursing & Personal Care Facilities
7. Educational Institutions: Elementary & Secondary Schools, College, Professional & Vocational Schools
8. Business Services: Services to Dwellings & Other Buildings (Janitorial), Services to Companies (Mailings, Packaging, Assembly, etc.)
9. General Merchandise Stores: Department Stores, Variety Stores, Miscellaneous General Merchandise Stores
10. Non-Profit Organizations (Volunteer Placements)

HEALTH CONDITIONS: Restricted Health Conditions:

- Use of inhalation-assistive devices
- Colostomy/ileostomy
- Need for fecal impaction removal, enemas, or suppositories
- Use of indwelling urinary catheters
- Staph or other serious, communicable infections
- Insulin-dependent diabetes
- Wounds (Stage 1 or 2 dermal ulcer or an unhealed, surgically closed incision or wound)
- Gastronomy (feeding, hydration, and care)
- Tracheostomies
- Clients with metered-dose inhalers and dry powder inhalers
- Clients who require oxygen

- Clients who rely upon others to perform all activities of daily living (ADL's)
  Bathing
  Dressing
  Toiletiing
  Transferring
  Eating
  Continence

- Clients with incontinence
- Clients with contractures
- Naso-gastric and naso-duodenal tubes
- Active, communicable TB
- Conditions that require 24-hour nursing care and monitoring
- Any other condition or care requirements which would require the facility to be licensed as a health facility as defined by Sections 1202 and 1250 of the Health and Safety Code

Universal Precaution

PROCEDURE	WASH	WEAR
DAY TO DAY INTERACTIONS	X	X
SHOWERINNG/BATHING, TOOTH BRUSHING, MISCELLANEOUS ORAL HYGIENE	X	X
MENSTRUAL CARE	X	X
FIRST AID	X	X
CHANGING LINENS/LAUNDRY	X	X
CLEANING UP TOILETING ACCIDENTS/VOMIT	X	X
TAKING RECTAL TEMPERATURE OR ADMINISTERING ENEMAS/SUPPOSITORIES	X	X
SHAVING WITH DISPOSABLE BLADE RAZORS	X	X
APPLYING TOPICAL MEDICATIONS	X	X
DISPENSING ORAL MEDICATIONS	X	X
COLLECTING URINE OR BM UNIVERSAL PRECAUTIONS	X	X

TO PREVENT TRANSMISSION OF BLOOD BORNE DISEASE

General Information

Many potentially communicable diseases go unrecognized so universal precautions (barrier precautions) should be taken routinely regardless of the known or unknown diagnosis of an individual when contact with blood or body fluids is anticipated.

All direct care staff (persons whose activities hands on contact with clients) should routinely use appropriate barrier precautions to prevent skin and mucous membrane exposure when contact with blood or other body fluids of any client is anticipated. Disposable gloves should be worn for touching blood and body fluids, mucous membranes or non-intact skin of all clients, for handling items or surfaces soiled with blood or body fluids. Staff should be aware of the potential for transmission of disease to client, client staff and client to client.

Techniques

Hand washing before and after contact with each client is the most effective way or preventing and controlling the spread of infection.

Hand washing should be done when:
- Arriving and leaving work;
- Between each direct contact with a client;
- Before and after use of disposable gloves;
- When hands are dirty;
- After handling soiled equipment and soiled linens;
- Preparing or serving meals;
- Preparing and dispensing medications;
- After using the bathroom for self and or client.

Essential of hand washing:
- Running water;
- Rub/scrub hands together;
- Cleansing agent such as soap or detergent (liquid soap preferred);
- Paper towels that are conveniently available.

Hand washing procedures:
- Remove watch and jewelry;
- Expose the forearms;
- Turn on water to a comfortable temperature;
- Scrub vigorously with soap and running water for at least 30 seconds, with special care to areas between fingers, around nails and forearms;
- Rinse thoroughly with water;
- Dry hands thoroughly with paper towels and discard paper towels in covered, lined trash container.

Gloves should be worn when assisting client with:
- Bathing or cleaning the rectal or genital areas;
- Giving mouth care;
- Shaving with a disposable blade razor;
- Cleaning toilets;
- Cleaning up urine, stool or vomit
- Menstrual care and disposal of sanitary pads;
- Performing wound care.

Gloves should be changed after direct contact with each client. Hands should be washed immediately after gloves are removed. If a glove is torn during use, remove glove and replace with a new glove. Gloves should always be worn when staff have open wounds or rashes on their hands.

General purpose utility gloves (rubber household gloves) may be used for housekeeping chores involving potential contact with blood, utility gloves may be decontaminated and re-used should be discarded if they are peeling, cracked or discolored, or if they have punctures, tears, or other evidence of deterioration. Disposable gloves should not be re-used.

Daily Reminders of Universal Precautions

Bathroom:

Bathrooms that are shared with should be cleaned and disinfected routinely with disinfectant diluted with water. Wash tubs/showers between each client use with spray bottle of disinfectant diluted with water. Gloves should be used when cleaning bathrooms. Toilet brushes should be soaked in disinfectant between uses and be replaced as needed. Dispose of urine, stool and vomit immediately. Dirty water used for mopping up the floor should not be disposed of in the sink where food is prepared.

Laundry:

All soiled linen should be handled as little as possible. Clothing or bed covers soiled with fecal matter, urine or blood should be washed separately and staff should wear gloves when handling these contaminated linens.

Personal Care:

Each clients needs own hygiene items: tooth brush, brush comb, and razor (if used). These items are not to be shared and need to be stored separately. Tooth brushes need to be changed frequently. Disposable gloves must be worn for all mouth care. Staff should change gloves after each client.

PRESSURE SORE

INCIDENTAL MEDICAL SERVICES
AREAS AFFECTING PROGRAM DESCRIPTION

1. If a client is to receive services and has a restricted health condition, the needs and services plan must include the restricted health condition care plan and the licensee shall involve the placement or referral agency, if any, in the development of the plan.

2. Prior to accepting a client who relies upon others to perform all activities of daily living, a needs and services plan must include an agreement, signed by the regional center, to review the client's care at least once a month.

3. The Home must identify all clients who have a Restricted Health Care Condition.

4. Whenever a client who relies on others to perform all activities of daily living is present, staffing shall be maintained as required by the regional center but not less than one direct care staff to three clients.

5. If the Home chooses to provide services to a client with a restricted health condition, a restricted health condition care plan shall be developed as part of the needs and services plan The plan shall document all parties involved in the development of the plan, the client, client's authorized representative, if any, client's physician or designee, and regional center representative(s);

   - Include a date specified by the client's physician or designee when the plan must be reviewed by all parties involved in development of the plan; and

   - Include a signed statement from the regional center representative that he/she has reviewed and approved the plan and will monitor the implementation of the plan.

6. Whenever a client of the regional center who relies upon others to perform all activities of daily living is present, staffing shall be maintained as specified by the regional center.

NEEDS AND SERVICES PLAN

Prior to admission, the Home shall determine whether the facility's program can meet the prospective client's service needs. If the client is to be admitted and has no restricted health condition(s) as specified in Section 80092, no later than 30 days after admission, the licensee shall complete a written Needs and Services Plan that must include:

(1). The client's desires and background and formal supports, obtained from the client's family or his/her authorized representative, if any, regarding the following:

(A). Admission to the facility

(B). Medical information including primary physician, health problems and medical history, prescribed medications and their strength, quantity required and purpose.

(C). Mental and Emotional functioning

(D). Functional limitations including physical impairments or concerns. The licensee may use Section 80069.2 for assistance.

(E). Specific service needs, if any

(F). Scheduled days of attendance.

(G). Transportation arrangements.

(H). If the client is to be admitted, and has a restricted health condition as specified in Section 80092(c) then, the licensee shall develop the Needs and Services Plan prior to admission.

RESTRICTED HEALTH CARE PLAN

Procedures for Accepting a Consumer

When a resident requires Restricted Conditions, the staff shall fill up this form:

For restricted conditions: (please explain each item in detail)

1. What is the condition?

2. What is the stability of the condition?

3. Describe the specific care needed.

4. How often is care needed for the condition?

5. Provide the name and title of the licensed professional medical person to provide the care.

6. If the assistance or care does not constantly require a licensed professional person to provide services, the Home shall provide the name(s) of direct care/program staff who have been trained by the licensed professional medical person.

7. In the event of an emergency, the Facility will notify what persons; please provide names and telephone numbers.

8. How often will the plan be reviewed?

    1. Document whether or not the plan meets the scope of medical practice requirements.

    2. Plan shall be prepared, completed, signed, and dated by a health care medical professional.

Romwell Martinez Sabeniano, MBA.HCM

(Sample Form)

Date:

To Whom It May Concern:

This letter is to establish the stability of (client name) _____ _____. This condition remains chronic and stable. This stability should allow him to begin attending a day program to enhance his general functional skills and social interaction.

He will require feeding and hydration one time per day via his g-tube while at day program. This service will be provided by the day program LVN. He is unable to perform this ask for himself due to severe mental retardation and cerebral palsy. In the event of an emergency, the staff will notify (Facility Name)_____ at (address) _____ followed by QMRP, _____ _ at (phone)_____. If determined to be necessary, 911 will be called for emergency care followed by calling above persons.

_____
Signature and Title

Date: _____

_____
Print Name

CERTIFICATION

I AGREE THAT (Facility Name)_____ for the (client population)_____ will provide services to (client name)_____ and agree to comply and cooperate with all requirements necessary in the Individual Health Care Plan. I also understand that (Facility Name)_____ provides only non-medical care and, in the event of emergency, I will be contacted as soon as possible after 911 has been called if deemed necessary by (Facility Name) _____ Facility.

_____   _____
Facility Name   Placement Agency

_____
Signature & Title Date

_____
Signature & Title Date

Romwell Martinez Sabeniano, MBA.HCM

Date

To Whom It May Concern:

I have reviewed, approved, and agreed to monitor the implementation of the Individual Health Care Plan for (Client Name)_____ _____. I will monitor the progress quarterly with further checkups if any emergency should arise.

_____
Placement Agency

_____
Signature & Title   Date

_____
Print Name

ADMISSION AGREEMENT ADDENDUM

I, AS CONSUMER/CLIENT REPRESENTATIVE, AGREE TO COMPLY WITH THE individual Health Care Plan developed by (Facility Name) _____ for (Client Name) _____. I also agree that _____ will attend (Facility Name) _____ five days per week from 8:30 a. m. to 2:30 p. m. with transportation being provided to and from home by (Facility Name) _____.

_____
Facility Name Date

_____ _____
Signature & Title Date

_____
Print Name

Romwell Martinez Sabeniano, MBA.HCM

FUNCTIONAL ASSESSMENT

Client Name_____

DOB:_____

UCI: _____Soc. Sec. No: _____

(Client)_____has a diagnosis of severe mental retardation and cerebral palsy. He has no apparent hearing or vision loss. He does not have the ability to communicate/express his wants and needs verbally or by movement. He is non-ambulatory due to cerebral palsy.

(Client)_____is unable to perform any self help skills, including bathing, dressing, hygiene, toileting or feeding. He is unable to reposition himself or sit up without support. He is unable to properly his wheelchair by himself.

(Client)_____currently receive Neurontin 300mg two times per day; Dilantin 50mg in a. m. and 100 mg. In p. m.; and Reglan 20 mg in p. m.

He has no known mental health deficits. His socialization skills are limited due to mental retardation. This also affects his cognitive functioning skills which are extremely limited. He has no abusive behaviors. He does not have the ability to manage his own finances.

INDIVIDUAL HEALTH CARE PLAN NOTE (Form)

(Client)_____ will be fed via his g-tube. His needs will be met according to acceptable guidelines. He will be fed one time per day at program with attends changed three times per day (he is incontinent). While client is unable to effectively communicate his wants and needs utilizing conventional methods (verbalization/ expressions), we will ensure that all staff are trained to identify needs/wants trough observation and familiarization with clients current methods of communications as reported by group home staff.

(Client)_____frowns and/or cry when he is uncomfortable. When all efforts to make comfortable are unsuccessful, contact numbers will be called. Emergency numbers are listed on the vital sheet kept in his chart. The emergency numbers will be contacted for medical and non-medical emergencies should the need arise.

(Client)_____will be repositioned in his wheelchair every _____ while at day program. Feeding and changing will occur at _____ by staff members. His feeding and all medical needs will be handled by the LVN and emergency contacts.

Romwell Martinez Sabeniano, MBA.HCM

Training Provided for Care Clients (Evaluation Form)

Client Name:_____

Staff will be trained to care for (Client)_____in the following manner by an LVN:

1. Staff will be trained to lift and transfer him to and from bed and changing table.

2. Staff will be trained to wash hands and face, brush teeth and hair according to (Client) _____ preference.

3. Staff will be trained how to communicate with Client _____, using his method of communications (smiles / frowns).

4. Staff will be trained to observe (Client)_____ for signs and symptoms of distress using his method of communication discomfort (crying, squirming in chair).

5. Instructors will be trained as to what activities (Client) _____ prefers to participate in and how to ascertain what activity he wishes to participate in.

PROGRAM DESIGN ADDENDUM

GASTROSTOMIES

Angel Care Home we will be caring for consumers with Gastrostomies. The care of the gastronomy will be provided by the LVN on duty. All G-tube feedings and care will be handled by the LVN, who will assure that g-tube is properly in place prior to initiating feedings, and assure that stoma area is clean and dry upon completion of feeding. The LVN will also be checking for signs or symptoms of distress, and immediately report any abnormalities to Registered Nurse (RN) or family members.

Client/consumers requiring g-tube feedings and care will be following the same programming schedule as other consumers in the program. The LVN will feed consumer via the g-tube while seated at the table with others so allow for the social interaction with other peers and staff members.

In the event of an emergency (i.e., the g-tube falling out), the RN or family member will be called immediately and provide us with further instructions. If deemed acceptable, the RN will come to the program and handle emergency situation.

TOTAL CARE

Staff will be trained as to how to provide total care for the consumer. They will be trained on how to change and observe for skin breakdown, how to handle if occurs, reposition to correct, and comfortable positions provided by the home, how to communicate using methods provided by the home, how to have client/consumer participate in programming activities according to preferences. Staff will also learn how to monitor for signs and symptoms of distress or discomfort according to Individual Health Care Plan and how to handle if any signs or symptoms are exhibited. In addition to this, they will be trained how to handle a situation should emergency intervention be required (i.e. 911), other than LVN, RN,

DOCUMENTATION OF TRAINING IN PERSONNEL FILES

Staff will be in serviced by LVN In all areas of total care for consumer as specified in 80077.2. They will be required to sign in on an in-service sheet that will then be photocopied and placed in their personnel files maintained in the Personnel/Payroll office at (Facility Name) _____.

REGISTER OF CLIENTS (Form)

We have_____ master books with vital sheets of all client/consumers in care at (Facility Name)_____ These books are located in the _____. This also serves as the register for client/consumers with restricted health conditions. These consumers have a vital sheet in these books that lists the restricted health conditions which are applicable to them.

FUNCTIONAL CAPABILITIES ASSESSMENT

NAME: FACILITY:

BATHING:
A. Does not bathe or shower self
B. Performs some bathing or showering tasks
C. Bathe or showers self independently

CONTINENCE:
A. No bowel and/or bladder control
B. Some bowel and/or bladder control
C. Use of assertive devices, such as catheter
Comments:_____
D. Complete bowel and/or bladder control

DRESSING:
A. Does not dress self
B. Puts on some clothing by self
C. Dresses self completely
Comments:_____

EATING:
A. Does not feed self.
B. Feeds self with assistance from another person
C. Feeds self completely
Comments:_____

GROOMING:
A. Does not tend to own personal hygiene
B. Tends to some personal hygiene tasks
C. Tends to own personal hygiene
Comments:_____

VISION:
A. Severe/profound impairment
B. Mild/moderate impairment
C. No vision impairment
Comments:_____

TOILETING:
A. Not toilet trained
B. Does not toilet self
C. Goes to toilet by self
Comments:_____

HEARING:
A. Severe/profound loss
B. Mild/moderate impairment
C. No hearing loss
Comments: _____

TRANSFERRING:
A. Unable to move in and out of a bed or chair
B. Needs assistance to transfer
C. Is able to move in and out of a bed or chair
Comments: _____

COMMUNICATION:
A. Does not express nonverbally
B. Does not express verbally
C. No hearing loss
Comments:_____

REPOSITIONING:
A. Unable to reposition
B. Repositions from side to side
C. Repositions from front to back and back to front
Comments: _____

CLOWN PARTY	COUNTY FAIR
WESTERN PARTY	CIRCUS PARTY
INDOOR BEACH PARTY	NAUTICAL PARTY
NEWPAPER PARTY	PIONEER PARTY
PUZZLE PARTY	SCAVENGER HUNT
PARTY	
HILLBILLY BASH	WINTER WONDERLAND A
MAGIC BANQUET	BREAKFAST IN THE YARD
SUPER BOWL PARTY	BARNYARD BASH
CANDY PULL	FASHION SHOW
HAWAIIAN HOLIDAY	HOLLYWOOD PARTY
MUSIC PARTY	PUPPET SHOW
PIRATE PARTY	GRANDPARENT PARTY
NEW YEARS EVE PARTY	ARBOR DAY PARTY
VALENTINE'S DAY PARTY	CUPID'S CARNIVAL OF HEARTS
GROUND HOG DAY	SADIE HAWKINS DAY PARTY
SAINT PATRICK'S DAY PARTY	SPRING PARTY
APRIL FOOL'S DAY PARTY	EASTER PARTY
MAY DAY PARTY	MOTHER'S DAY PARTY
MEMORIAL DAY	4TH OF JULY
FATHER'S DAY	PATRIOTIIC PARTY
GYPSY PARTY	COLUMBUS DAY PARTY
HALOWEEN PARTY	HALOWEEN CARNIVAL
THANKSGIVING PARTY	VETERAN;S DAY PARTY
CHRISTMAS DAY PARTY	CHRISTMAS CONCERT
CHRISTMAS PARADE	CHRISTMAS EVE

MONEY RAISING ACTIVITIES

APRON BAZAAR	CHRISTMAS BOTIQUE
WHITE ELEPHANT AUCTION	GARAGE SALE
RUMMAGE SALE	FAVORITE RECIPE BOOK
BAKE SALE	CHILI SUPPER
PANCAKE BREAKFAST	PIE SOCIAL
SPAGHETTI BREAKFAST	HOT DOG STAND

GOALS OF A RECREATIONAL PROGRAM

To provide varied opportunities for the constructive use of leisure time. To provide pleasure and creative satisfaction, and to serve as a form of personal achievement and personality development. To promote healthful physical involvement, and to prevent further physical deterioration because of disuse. To aid in the restoration of the consumers' physical, mental, and social functions. To enhance the social independence of the individual and give him satisfying group experiences in a well rounded schedule of activity.

GENERAL POLICIES OF AN ACTIVITY PROGRAM

1. The activities coordinator is designated as being responsible for the planning and development of all consumers' activities.

2. The activities program will be satisfied and equipped to meet the needs and interests of each consumer.

3. The activity coordinator shall supervise the recruitment and training of all volunteers.

4. The activity coordinator shall aid in the development of a consumers.

5. The activities program shall provide a variety of activities related to current consumers interests.

6. Be notified of all Admissions.

7. Work in cooperation with nursing, dietary and services departments.

8. Be informed of precautions relative to consumers whose condition would restrict their activities.

9. Conduct in-service training programs relating to consumers activities.

10. That safety procedures related activities and consumers' protection are known by staff and volunteers.

ASSESSMENT/EVALUATION

The Administrator together with the Nurse shall have primary responsibility for evaluation of planned activities.

1. Facility shall keep on file an activity interest assessment form for each consumer.

2. Facility shall keep on file an individual consumer activity plan.

3. Facility shall keep on file document forms for activity schedules, consumers participation and evaluations.

4. Facility shall have a consumer/family suggestion box.

ARTHRITIS

Arthritis is an inflammation or swelling of a joint. In most case, it occurs gradually. Most forms are chronic, lasting for years. In seniors, the two most common forms are Osteoarthritis and Rheumatoid. The underlying cause of Arthritis is not known, but the effect on the joints and pain can be substantial.

The consumer might complain about aching, swelling, stiffness (especially in the morning or after a nap), and pain of various degrees. Medical science has developed some good medications to combat Arthritis. The success of these medications varies from consumer to consumer. It is imperative to keep the weight. Exercise, diet, and adequate rest can help in keeping the symptoms at a minimum.

OSTEOARTHRITIS

The Most common form of Arthritis is Osteoarthritis. "Osteo" means bone, and "itis" means inflammation. This is a degenerative joint disease that produces stiffness or pain in the fingers or in weight bearing joints, such as knees, hips and the spine. Over 75 % of the Seniors in America are affected in one form or another by this disease.

RHEUMATOID ARTHRITIS

Rheumatoid Arthritis can affect almost all of the joints. Chronic inflammation will deform a joint by causing sticky adhesions. These adhesions will become scar tissue and eventually harden. The sufferer will go through periods of "flair ups", leaving more and more damage each time, if not arrested. Women are affected three times more frequently than men. The onset of the disease usually begins in the small joints in the hands and the feet.

ARTHRITTIS AND RELATED DISEASE

Chief Complaints:
Physical:
ACHING PAIN IN JOINTS
USE IS LIMITED   INFLAMED TISSUES
                         AROUND JOINTS
TIREDNESS   REDNESS
STIFFNESS   HEAT IN JOINT AREAS
SEVERE "FLAIR UPS" SHOULD ALWAYS BE REPORTED
TO THE PHYSICIAN

EMOTIONAL: Because this is usually a chronic disease, sufferers can display emotional symptoms such as depression, irritability, and helplessness. (See chronic Illness for more examples)

TIPS TO ASSIST A PERSON WITH ARTHRITIS AND RELATED DISEASES:

    a.   Have the attending physician diagnose the problem and follow-up. Make sure the consumer follows prescribed medication regimen.

    b.   Make sure the consumer is getting the proper diet, exercise and sleep. Encourage Range of Motion exercises.

c. Adapt the living necessities so that the consumer can cope as much for self as possible.

d. Make sure clothing is easily managed. Velcro can be put on instead of buttons. Make sure shoes and slippers fit properly and give adequate support. Adaptive eating equipment (WITH LARGE HANDLE OR PLATE GUARDS) can be utilized. Cut the consumer's meat in small bite size pieces.

Physical therapy as prescribed by the physician. The therapist can administer a heat treatment that can be helpful.

HOT SHOWERS OR BATHS CAN BE HELPFUL.

GOUT

Gout is caused by a defect in the uric acid. The body does not eliminate this waste product from the urine. Currently, the cause for this is unknown. Too much alcohol or Vitamin C can cause more acid in the urine; they should be avoided. Gout can cause pain and swelling in the joints and has periods of "flair ups" which cause a great deal of pain. Medications for prevention and acute attacks are often prescribed.

HIP FRACTURES AND REPLACEMENTS

Hip fractures are one of the most common type of fractures occurring in the elderly. The hip is a ball and socket joint. The fracture usually results from a fall. The fall may caused by tripping or misplaced footing but can occur, for example, from stepping off a curb or stair.

Osteoarthritis and Rheumatoid Arthritis can be extremely painful and severely affect the physical abilities of the sufferer. In these types of cases many times a hip replacement is performed.

If a hip is indicated, often the physician will recommend the person have physiotherapy treatment. The stronger the muscles and joint surrounding the hip are, the better the result will be from the surgery. The surgeon can replace the hip but not the muscles, tendons and ligaments.

Artificial components, a socket, ball and shaft make up the prostheses to replace the defected parts. The success is very high and the recovery rate is usually very good.

Physical and Occupational therapy can assist the consumer in returning to a normal level of functioning. Often, adaptive devices can help ease activities of daily living.

It is important for the consumer to understand they may not walk as well as they had expected to. The hip area will be sore. It will take time to establish strength in the hip. The Physician and Physical Therapist will determine whether a person will use a walker or crutches. Crutches are usually preferred when there are no other medical problems to consider because they allow for a normal walking pattern to be established.

At any time, even years later, a hip prosthesis can displace or become defective in some manner. It rarely happens, but it can occur. If a consumer complains about pain in the area, seek medical attention.

GASTROINTESTINAL DISORDERS

Gastrointestinal disorders are those illness or disease related to the digestive system. The most common examples affecting the elderly are as follows:

Constipation
Peptic Ulcers
Diverticulitis
Irritable Bowel Syndrome
Hemorrhoids

Diarrhea
Heartburn and Indigestion
Hiatus Hernia
Colitis

CONSTIPATION

Many seniors suffer from constipation due to their use of prescription medications like pain killers and over-the-counter medications such as constipation.

Constipation can be described as the inability and/or difficulty of passing a stool. The stool is usually hard and dry. Medication is usually tried to assist in the elimination process. If the stool is not successfully eliminated, an impaction can occur. Impaction is defined as a large amount of hard or soft stool usually in the large intestine, that the person is unable to pass. This can lead to a life threatening situation in which surgery may be required. An ASP (Appropriately Skilled Professional) can perform a rectal exam and contact the attending physician for orders to try an enema(s) or to physically remove the impaction.

SIGNS AND SYMPTOMS:

Physical Signs:	Symptoms:
Leaking grainy stool	Unable to eliminate and have constant urge
Distended	Pain in abdomen and rectum
Firm & tender abdomen	Nausea and loss of appetite
Low grade fever	Emotional distress

TIPS ON PREVENTION:

1. Have the consumer keep track daily of bowel activity
2. Proper Diet and exercise
3. Regular elimination schedule (45 minutes after a meal works well)

Fiber can help in the prevention of constipation. Whole grain cereals, fresh fruits and vegetables, fruit juices and whole wheat bread are good sources of fiber. Prunes and prune juice are healthy – natural laxatives. Many people testify to hot or warm prune juice being extremely effective. Other types of laxatives such as Castor Oil, Bisacodyl, Ducolax, Milk of Magnesia and Cascara.

DIARRHEA

Certain medications can cause diarrhea, but diarrhea is most often caused by an infection or food allergies. Diarrhea is frequent elimination of watery stools. Stress can also be prime factor in causing diarrhea. Rigorous cramping can occur before and during a diarrhea attack.

If food is not properly stored, prepared or handled, food poisoning can occur. This is easily prevented by proper training of the dietary staff, posted policies and procedures regarding sanitation, cooking, storage and handling of food items.

If food allergy is suspected, the attending physician can perform tests to investigate further and advice to proper dieting.

SIGNS AND SYMPTOMS

Physical:
Cramping	Urgency
Watery stool	Frequency
Flatulence	

HOW TO ASSIST:

Clear liquid diet (if you can't see through it, it's not clear liquid). As person improves, add: Rice Water, ripe banana, cream of wheat or rice, avoid fats & spicy foods, or over-the counter remedies. If the problem persists seek advise from the attending physician.

TAKE STEPS TO PREVENT DEHYDRATION. IF DEHYDRATION DOES OCCUR, CONTACT THE PHYSICIAN IMMEDIATELY OR SEEK IMMEDIATE MEDICAL ATTENTION.

PEPTIC ULCERS

Peptic ulcers are open areas in the lining of the upper intestines, stomach or esophagus. Due to an imbalance of the body's natural digestive aids, increased acids and enzymes can cause ulcers to develop. The pain can be severe and/or belching can occur. There are now several medications that can heal and improve an ulcer condition. Proper diet, reduced stress levels, and avoiding smoking can help prevent ulcers or reoccurrence.

BEWARE: SOME MEDICATIONS CAN CAUSE PEPTIC ULCERS

HEARTBURN AND INDIGESTION

Heartburn and indigestion occur when the stomach acids back up to the esophagus. Regurgitation can occur. If this is a chronic problem the consumer should be seen by the attending physician. Antacids should only be give per doctor's orders.

PREVENTIONS OF HEARTBURN AND INDIGESTION

1. Avoid acid and fatty foods.
2. Avoid carbonated and caffeinated drinks
3. Quit smoking
4. Cook fruits and vegetables
5. Reduce stress

DIVERTICULITIS

Diverticuli are small sac-like pockets formed on the large intestine wall. This is an exceedingly common disease in the elderly. Many persons with diverticuli do not have any symptoms. Others, unfortunately, have many. Diverticulitis is the inflammation of the diverticuli. This occurs when the sac-like pockets are filled with feces, seeds or nuts. The symptoms are pain, diarrhea and/or constipation, vomiting and nausea. If a consumer is suffering from these symptoms, he should see his physician. As an ongoing treatment for diverticulitis, high fiber diets are often recommended.

HERNIA

A hernia is defined as an abnormal protrusion of an organ through a weak wall in the body cavity. The most common type of hernia occurs in the groin area.

A hiatus hernia is the stomach protruding partially into the chest cavity because of the hiatus (the opening in the diaphragm) being too wide. This condition can cause heartburn, indigestion and regurgitation.

PRECAUTIONS FOR HERNIA SUFFERS:

1. Eat slowly and chew food completely
2. Drink liquids apart from mealtimes
3. Avoid carbonated drinks
4. Avoid over-eating
5. Don't lay down immediately after a meal; it is best to wait two hours before retiring. Keep the head of the bed slightly elevated.
6. Don't wear items too tight in the stomach area.

IRRITABLE BOWEL SYNDROME

Irritable Bowel Syndrome is one of the "Twentieth Century" disease. Sufferers have symptoms of cramps and diarrhea caused by spasms in the large intestines. This is also termed spastic colon, and nervous bowel. Inflammation of the colon (colitis) can occur.

When this illness becomes chronic, ulcers can occur and complicate the condition. Stress, diet, and food allergy may cause or contribute to irritable bowel syndrome.

However, there is no concrete proof as to the actual cause. In severe case, anticholinergic and sedative types of medications may be prescribed.

HEMORRHOIDS

Hemorrhoids may occur internally or externally in the rectum/anus area. Pain, burning, itching, and a small amount of bleeding can occur. Chronic constipation or pressure on the veins of the rectum cavity will create hemorrhoids. A good way or pressure to describe hemorrhoids is varicose veins of the rectum. Other contributing causes are excessive use of laxatives, obesity, liver disorders, and rectal tumors.

High fiber diets will make the elimination process easier, thus relieving pressure on the rectum. In severe cases, surgery may be necessary. The attending physician may prescribe sits baths, suppositories or topical ointments. If suppositories are needed and the consumer is unable to do self care an ASP (Approximately Skilled Professional). Can assist.

RESPIRATORY DISEASES

EMPHYSEMA

Cigarette smoking is the number one cause of emphysema. Seldom is emphysema inherited. It's development begins early in life, but the symptoms will appear in the later years.
Emphysema is a lung disease in which the alveoli (air sacks in the lungs) become damaged to the point where they can no longer hold air. The emphysema sufferer will be short of breath.

Edema and chronic bronchitis will often accompany emphysema. A person with this disorder may develop a persistent chronic cough and a wheeze.

There is no cure for Emphysema; treatments only help relieve some of the symptoms. The damaged lung tissue cannot be replaced. Treatment includes restricting the sodium intake in the diet. As the condition becomes more severe, the person will have to use a canula and oxygen equipment.

ASTHMA

Asthma is an illness that usually begins in early childhood, but can occur at any age. It has a tendency to clear up by the early adult years.

The most familiar kind of Asthma is Bronchial Asthma. There are two basic types of Bronchial Asthma. Extrinsic, is the type that is brought on by an allergic reaction like hay fever. Intrinsic is the second type and usually comes later in life and is often brought only by a respiratory tract infection, emotional problems stress, anxiety, and the like.

Asthma attacks can vary from mild discomfort to respiratory failure. The main symptoms are wheezing, shortness of breath, a dry cough, and a tight feeling in the chest.
Preventive measures can be taken will good results; however, there is no cure for Asthma at this time. Immunotherapy can be performed but its success is limited. The most commonly used drugs on the market today are prophylactic (preventive) drugs and inhaled corticosteroid drugs.

PLEURISY

Pleurisy is an inflammation of the membrane lining in the lungs. Viral Pneumonia is one possible cause. Pleurisy causes sharp pains to occur with every breath. Pleurisy can usually be effectively treated with antibiotics.

PNEUMONIA

Pneumonia is an infection caused by viruses and/or bacteria, involving the membrane lining. The two main kinds are Lobar Pneumonia and Bronchopneumonia. The inflammation in bronchopneumonia takes hold in the bronchi and bronchiolus (air passages into the lungs) but then spreads and may eventually involve both lungs.

The symptoms include fever, chills, shortness of breath, chest pains when breathing, an increased amount of sputum that is usually green or yellow-green in color, and pleurisy. Tylenol or Aspirin (if allowed) will help reduce the fever. Antibiotics and/or antifungal will usually care Pneumonia.

PULMONARY OBSTRUCTION

The common type of pulmonary obstruction is pulmonary embolism (clot). The embolism is a blood clot that has broken free from its place of origin, usually from inside a leg. The embolism will travel through the bloodstream until it encounters an area narrower than itself. Most often, this will be in the heart or lungs.

The symptoms include dizziness, sharp chest pains when breathing, rapid pulse shortness of breath, and coughing up blood.

The use of thrombolytic drugs can be an effective treatment. If the embolism is small enough in size, then anticoagulants can be used to dissolve it. Surgery may be needed if the embolus (clot) is very large.

DIABETES

There are two types of diabetes. Type 1 is insulin-dependent and Type 2 is non-insulin-dependent. Often, they are referred to as "juvenile-onset", insulin-dependent, or "adult-onset", non-insulin-dependent. Both types of diabetes can occur at any time, but usually begin at the age associated it.

Diabetes is a result of a defect in the metabolism of sugar (glucose). Sugar and starches (carbohydrates) are changed into glucose and enter the bloodstream. Once a person develops diabetes, it is usually a chronic disease, lasting for the rest of his life.

Type1, insulin-dependent diabetes, usually starts during childhood and is caused by an insufficient production of, or a complete failure to produce insulin. Insulin is normally produced by the pancreas. It is a hormone which regulates the body's use of glucose. If the person's body produces too little, or none at all, they must have insulin daily (sometimes several times a day). If they do not get the insulin, the body becomes hyperglycemic – TOO MUCH SUGAR! This can be extremely dangerous, possibly fatal.

Type2, non-insulin-dependent diabetes, is usually controlled by diet and/or oral medication. The onset is usually during middle age. It is more common in women than in men. About a third of Type 2 diabetics can be successfully treated by diet without any medication. If the person follows the diet prescribed by the physician, gets rest, and gets plenty of exercise, they may be able to live medication "free".

With both types of diabetics, monitoring should be done. An ASP (Appropriately Skilled Professional) from local home health service agency can monitor the consumer and Medi-Care usually pays for it. Routine doctor visits should be attended. Always remember that the consumer needs to give himself the insulin injection, or it can be done by an SP. If the ASP performs the service, make sure you keep the ASP's name, plan, and services accurately documented.

HYPERGLYCEMIA

Hyperglycemia will occur when there is too much sugar (glucose) in the blood stream. The accumulation is usually a gradual process. Often you can observe signs or symptoms which indicate the sugar is on the rise.

Signs and symptoms:

Excessive Hunger
    Frequent Urination
    Weakness
    Muscle Pain
    Abdominal Pain or Vomiting
    Deep Rapid Breathing
    Confusion
    Emotional Changes

Prevention:

Proper Diet
Exercise
Routine blood tests for glucose level

HYPOGLYCEMIA

This is the term used for low blood sugar. This can rapidly lead to a critical condition or death. It is caused primarily by either too much insulin, infection, a lack of food or excessive exercise.

Symptoms:

- Weakness
- Sweaty
- Tremors & Shaking

- Headaches
- Hunger
- Personality Changes

Hypoglycemia can result in seizure or coma.
IF UNCONSCIOUS, CALL 911

If conscious, seek immediate medical attention. The ASP or consumer should check blood sugar level. If the sugar level is 40 or lower, have the consumer consume one of the following:

4oz to 6oz	Apple juice
4oz to 6oz	Orange juice
4oz to 6oz	Soft Drink (not diet)
1 Tablespoon	Grape Jelly
1 Tablespoon	Corn Syrup

RE-CHECK BLOOD SUGAR LEVEL AFTER 5 MINUTES; IF STILL LOW, REPEAT WITH A SECOND DOSE.

CALL ATTENDING PHYSICIAN WITH REPORT AND RESULTS.

INCONTINENCE

Incontinence can be contributed to illness, a physical problem or medication. Many seniors have a minor incontinence problem of leakage. This is easily managed by a disposable undergarment like Depends, Attends, incontinent pad or generic equivalent.

Incontinence is humiliating for most seniors. Often, they may withdraw from social interaction to avoid embarrassment. Wetting of clothing and hiding of undergarments may occur as the consumer may be too disconcerted to let the care provider know.

About 1 in 10 persons over the age of 65 has a problem with some degree of urinary incontinence. Coughing or laughing can put pressure on the bladder and cause leakage.

It is essential that a record of when, how long, how much and other pertinent information be kept to establish a pattern, if any, and to provide the Appropriately Skilled Professional (ASP) a basis for diagnosis.

Some consumers can be retrained by the ASP to control their bladders. Being sure the consumer urinates every 2 hours is usually the first step in establishing a routine. The consumer might be instructed to do some exercises to improve muscle tone. Occasionally, a doctor may prescribe a medication to help control incontinency.

TIPS ON INCONTINENCY

1. Visit a doctor make sure the consumer does not have an infection.

2. Make sure the toilet is easily accessible and nearby. Commodes may be used at night if cleaned promptly and stored away during the day.

3. Encourage the intake of fluids, especially clear ones like water.

4. Remind the consumer to go to the restroom.

5. Make sure garments are easily removed.

PROSTATE DISEASE

Elderly men should be checked annually for prostate disease. A rectal exam can be done in the physician's office during a routine visit. The prostate is a small organ about the size of a walnut. It is located next to the bladder (where urine is stored) and surrounds the urethra (the canal through which urine passes out of the body). Because of the close proximity to the urethra, an enlarged prostate can make urination difficult.

Acute prostatitis is the inflammation of the prostate resulting from a bacterial infection. It can usually be treated successfully with antibiotics. When the infection reoccurs continuously, antibiotics may be used for 3 months. Often the condition clears up by itself, but symptoms may last a long time.

Benign prostatic hypertrophy (BPH) is an enlargement of the prostate. It is caused by small noncancerous tumors that grow inside the prostate. It is not known what causes these growths, but they may be related to hormone changes with aging.

An enlarged prostate may, eventually, obstruct the urethra and cause difficulty urinating. Dribbling after urination and the urge to urinate frequently are common symptoms. In rare cases, the consumer may be unable to urinate. In severe cases, surgery may be necessary to remove the overgrown or tumor areas of the prostate.

URINARY TRACT INFECTIONS

Urinary tract infections usually effect the kidney, bladder or prostate organs. Symptoms like painful urination, burning or frequent urination, fever and groin pain occur. Incontinence can be a sign urinary tract infection. A urine analysis is usually performed to detect the infection and cause.

In cystitis, the bladder is inflamed from bacterial causes. Obstruction, mostly in men, can also lead to cystitis. The onset is often sudden. The physician will usually prescribe an antibiotic and a lot of fluids. After about 10 days the infection has typically abated.

Other problems like a defective ureter or pyelitis are causes of urinary tract infection. Medical attention should always be sought.

Urinary tract infections are treatable disorders; however, if left untreated, chronic infections can lead to permanent damage. Usually surgery or other extreme medical procedures can help to successfully overcome the problem.

It is important to follow up with a repeat Urinary Analysis to ensure the infection is gone.

HEART DISEASE

There are many types of cardiovascular diseases. About half of all Americans develop some form of heart disease. Heart disease can be hereditary. The age and sex of a person can increase the chances of heart disease. These include reducing high blood pressure, avoiding or quitting smoking, and lowering blood cholesterol.

ANGINA

This is the most common form of heart disease in adults and seniors. There are two basic types of angina. Classic angina results from arteriosclerosis (hardening of the arteries). Arterioclerosis occurs as fatty deposits develop and clogging transpires. This may develop over many years. When the artery is clogged, "angina", a temporary pain in the chest occurs. Variant angina can strike from a spasm or constriction of the coronary artery. When the blood flow is cut off as a result of the spasm or constriction, "angina", a pain very similar to that of classic angina occurs.

Unstable angina is term used to describe the angina resulting from both types of angina, separately occurring at various times. If the consumer uses nitroglycerine, the standard is 1 every 5 minutes up to 3 doses. If no relief occurs, call an ambulance.

ARRHYTHMIAS

Impulse beats of the heart occur 60 to 100 times a minute. The number of beats per minute is called the heart rate. The heart rate can increase with exercise or stressful situations and decrease with sleep and relaxation. Arrhythmias are distinctive irregular beats of the heart rate, originating from the heart. Many people experience minor irregular beats from time to time but distinctive arrhythmias should be taken seriously.

HYPERTENSION

Hypertension can be defined as too much tension on the blood vessel walls. The primary cause of hypertension is unknown, yet many factors can increase the chance of developing it. Medical sciences has sufficiently proven that smoking, obesity, and excessive salt usage can increase the chance of developing high blood pressure. Many medications are successful in keeping the blood pressure within normal limits; these include Diuretics, Vasodialators, and Beta Blockers.

CONGESTIVE HEART FAILURE

Congestive heart failure (CHF) is caused from the heart's failure to pump blood. CHF typically develops gradually over a period of time. There are many treatments that can reduce the painful and disabling affects, but it left untreated, death can occur. When the pumping of the blood by the heart is reduced, the blood and oxygen supply to other parts of the body is decreased. The body functions will begin malfunctioning. Many symptoms can occur such as shortness of breath, swelling or water retention (edema) and rapid heart beat. Anemia, serious Vitamin B deficiency, Hyperactive Thyroid, and Bacterial Infections can also cause CHF.

Mediation can successfully treat the symptoms of CHF and the person can live a relatively normal life, but should maintain routine visits to the attending physician for monitoring.

It is further recommended that the consumer's weight be checked once a week. Specifically watch for the feet and ankles swelling. If the consumer has gained more than 5 pounds, the physician should be notified. It is important for the consumer to take the prescribed medication properly and follow a low sodium diet.

Other types of heart disease include the following:
ASHD
Heart Valve Disorders
Congenital Heart Defects
Bradycardia
Rheumatic Fever
Mitral Valve Prolapse
Pericarditis

STROKE

The American Heart Association offers the following statistics about stroke:

- Stroke is the third leading cause of death in the United Sates.

- There are approximately half a million new stroke cases each year.

- Of these, nearly 75% occur in persons 65 years or older.
- Strokes occur more frequently in men than in women.
- Most stroke victims survive.
- Twenty percent of stroke victims develop aphasia.

Stroke is a general term used to describe the interruption of blood flow to the brain. The amount of damage caused by the stroke will depend on the severity and the area affected. Most strokes are caused by a blood clot or hemorrhage. There are two common types of strokes: CVA Cerebral Vascular Accident and TIA Transient Ischemic Attack.

CVA – CEREBRAL VASCULAR ACCIDENT

When a cerebral vascular attack occurs, the damage is permanent. However, in time, some recovery may occur. Many older persons have hardening or narrowing of the arteries in the brain to one degree or another. This condition is called arteriosclerosis. High blood pressure is a prime factor in the development of arteriosclerosis. When the hardening or narrowing is substantial this can lead to the forming of clot. When this clot occurs the functions control by that area are partially or completely hindered. This type of stroke is called cerebral thrombosis and typically occurs during sleep.

Another type of clot is called an embolism. This usually is formed in the large arteries of the neck. When it breaks off, it is carried by the blood stream to the brain, causing a stroke termed cerebral embolism. This is common in persons suffering from a heart attack and most often happens when a person is awake.

CEREBRAL HEMORRHAGE

The most serious kind of stroke is called cerebral hemorrhage. This type kills approximately 75 to 90 percent of its victims.

Hemorrhage is bleeding, cerebral is brain, cerebral hemorrhage is bleeding in the brain. The bleeding results when an aneurysm bursts, interrupts the blood flow and spills out onto the surrounding blood cells causing even more damage. This type usually occurs during the waking hours and has other symptoms like headache, vomiting and loss of consciousness.

TIA's - TRANSIENT ISCHEMIC ATTACK

This type of stroke is commonly called a mini-stroke. It can cause permanent damage with chronic reoccurrences. TIA's are a definite warning sign that something is amiss. Blood thinning and anti-clothing medications are often prescribed to prevent a stroke. TIA's symptoms include temporarily blurred vision, difficulties in verbal communication (speech, reading and writing), motor coordination, and dizzy spells.

PREVENTION SUGGESTION:

1. Reduce high blood pressure, and monitor regularly.
2. Eat a proper diet, avoid obesity.
3. Regularly exercise.
4. Medication therapy, if needed, as prescribed by the doctor.

UNDERSTANDING APHASIA

Understanding the aphasic person is the key to providing proper care. Sometimes the aphasic person is thought to be confused, but that is not the case. Aphasia is the most common type of language disorder in adults. It is usually caused by a cerebrovascular accident (CVA, or stroke). A stroke is an interruption in the flow of blood to the brain. In aphasia, this interruption happens in the area of the brain that control speech. Over half of the persons suffering from a stroke have a degree of this speech disorder. Head injury or trauma can also cause aphasia.

The brain is separate into two large globes. The right and left cerebral hemisphere comprise the "thinking" areas of the brain. The cerebral hemispheres sit on top of the cerebellum, a smaller globe that extends to form the spinal cord.

Speech is controlled by the left hemisphere of the brain, and injury to this area results in aphasia. Between one-third and one-half off all left-brain will produce some degree of aphasia.

TIPS ON COMMUNICATING WITH A PERSON WITH APHASIA:

1. Never rush the person, try to communicate in a calm atmosphere.
2. Use simple words and directions.
3. Give him/her plenty of time to talk and encourage him/her to talk.
4. Use eyes and no questions.
5. Give positive reinforcement.
6. Establish routines and consistency in activities of daily living.
7. If necessary, use a word or alphabet board.

Speech therapy may be covered under MEDI-CARE for up to a one-year period of time. Some home health services can provide speech therapy in consumer care.

DEALING WITH MEMORY PROBLEMS

1. Establish a fixed routine, whenever possible.
2. Keep messages short and clearly stated.
3. Give directions one step at a time.
4. Repeat training as often as necessary.
5. Use memory aides, like posters, with important information.
6. To help him/her remember his/her room, use familiar objects from his/hers home.
7. Have all staff, family, and friends repeat the same directions when training someone for a specific problem.

HEARING LOSS AND DEAFNESS

Many seniors suffer from hearing loss but few are totally deaf. As we grow older, the nerves (sound receptors) decrease in efficiency. The result is we hear less. Many times, ear wax builds up and block the ear from hearing clearly. In truly deaf people, there are physical changes in the middle ear. Infections, birth defects or injury to the middle ear can cause deafness or hearing loss.

We know that a good portion of what we hear is actually what we see. We read body language unconsciously. Have you ever heard someone tell you that a person only hears when he/she wants to? That may be due to the fact that when they want to, they are concentrating and paying attention to the body language. They may hear a little and see a lot which equals being able to understand.

Many hearing aid companies will provide free hearing tests to your consumers in order to sell their hearing aids. Unfortunately, hearing aids are not covered by Medi-Care and can be extremely costly.

When the consumer is visiting the Attending Physician, request that he/she check the consumer's ear and clean them, if necessary. If you have an ASP (Appropriately Skilled Professional) on staff, you may choose to have this service performed for your consumers on a regular basis.

Remember, persons with hearing disorders should be spoken to directly. Don't shout, but talk in a clear low-loud voice. Minimize the disruptive sounds when possible, like the TV and radio; shut the door, if possible.

A hearing aid is only good when it is used and adjusted properly. Usually, when a consumer first gets a hearing aid it is worn 1 to 2 hours a day. Most doctors recommend a gradual build up of use. We need to be patient with the consumer and give him assistance when needed.

TIPS ON CARING FOR HEARING AIDS:

A. Check the battery. Place the hearing aid in your hand and cover with your other hand; it should squeal if the battery is good. If the battery needs replacing, find the little latch to pull and replace the battery with the same type that is in it. These are usually found in any Drug Store.

B. Check setting. Often the consumer will have it too high or too low. If you are unable to adjust it comfortably for the consumer, have him see the Otorhinolaryngologist.

C. Check the ear mold portion and make sure it is clean. Never use alcohol for cleaning; it can cause cracks in the mold.
D. Have the consumer take the hearing aid out when sitting under a hair dryer.

Types of Hearing Aids:

A. Ear mold – most commonly used
B. Behind the Ear – very compact
C. Eyeglass hearing aid – used specifically for routing signals to the good ear.

PREVENTION OF BEDSORES (DECUBITI)

For Every hour it takes to cause a bedsore, 50 hours of treatment are needed to heal it. A bedsore can appear in a few hours. The skin can become red after 30 to 60 minutes of increased pressure. The inside area of a bedsore is more widespread than the outside area. In other words, it is much worse inside than it looks outside. Bedsores are caused by continued pressure on an area, which causes that area to have decreased circulation. Death of the tissue begins after two hours of pressure.

The best way to treat a bed sore is to prevent it. Licensing prohibits decubitus in consumer care facilities unless an exception has been granted.

OTHER CAUSES: PREVENTION

Urine or feces on skin   Keep consumer clean.
Bed wrinkles   Makes the linens smooth.
Dehydration   Encourage water and fluids
Damp skin   Pat completely dry after bathing
Soap (use only when necessary) Rinse soap off thoroughly

AREAS TO OBSERVE:

Back of head   Backbone
Shoulder blades   Buttocks

Elbows	Front of knees
Ankles	Inside of knees
Heels of feet	Leg braces, back braces, etc.

Paralyzed or contracted areas where skin meets skin.

NOTE: Bedsores can be prevented in these areas by padding.

ALZHEIMER'S DISEASE

Alzheimer's disease is a progressive condition where the brain and substance of the brain shrinks. In the elderly, it is estimated that 75% of dementia cases result from Alzheimer's; 30% of those 85 or older are affected.

The cause of Alzheimer's is unknown but there are several proposed theories. One theory is that Alzheimer's is caused by the effects of a chronic infection. Another is that Alzheimer's is brought on by toxic poisoning by a metal such as aluminum. There is known to be a reduced level of aceytlcholine and other brain chemicals in persons with Alzheimer.

Scientific findings have proven that Alzheimer's is a disease, not an inevitable consequence of old age. Alzheimer's can affect younger adults, but far less frequently than older persons. Recent studies indicated 10% to 20% percent of Alzheimer's cases might be inherited.

The onset of Alzheimer's Disease for the majority of persons suffering from this condition is in the mid 60's with death occurring within 7 to 10 years. A person with Alzheimer's eventually has decreased abilities for self care. This increases vulnerability to pneumonia and other infections which can lead to death.

At first, the individual with Alzheimer's disease experiences only minor, and almost imperceptible, symptoms that are often attributed to emotional upsets and other physical illnesses. Gradually, however, the person becomes more forgetful-particularly about recent events – and this may be reported by anxious relatives.

The person may neglect to turn off the stove, may misplace things, may recheck to see if a task was done, may take longer to complete a chore that was previously routine, or may repeat already answered questions. As the disease progresses, memory loss and changes in personality, mood, and behavior including confusion, irritability, restlessness, and agitation are likely to appear. Judgment, concentration, orientation, writing, reading, speech, motor behavior, and naming of objects may also be affected.

The pattern of care for persons with Alzheimer's disease is not unlike the long-term care required for many other adults with multiple chronic physical and mental impairments. In the early and middle stages of progressive dementia, relatives and friends provide most of the personal care necessary.

The same pattern often occurs when an older person has some other disease. In it's final and most debilitating stages, Alzheimer's disease often forces placement in a nursing home or long-term care institution. This can result from caregiver "burn-out", inability to provide the level of care needed or a combination of both. The same thing may happen in a family with an older member who has cancer, emphysema or some chronic disorder other than Alzheimer's.

A new brain-imaging technique, Positron Emission Tomography (PET), indicates differences in the brain metabolism of normal, depressed and demented persons. This work has shown that on the average, overall brain metabolism is normal in depressed persons is reduced 17 percent in persons with dementia due to blood circulation problems in the brain and is reduced 33 percent in Alzheimer's disease sufferers. Metabolic differences in particular brain regions were also found to follow distinct patterns in each type of case. Studies of these distinct patterns may provide useful data on why certain mental functions are lost inn Alzheimer's disease while other functions are spread.

The pace has accelerated dramatically in the search for an effective treatment for Alzheimer's disease. During the fast few years, several findings that may prove highly significant were reported. First, studies with cholinergic agent lecithin demonstrated that clinically modest, but reliable, brief improvements in memory can be produced in some patients with Alzheimer's disease.

Early findings from studies with lecithin combined with the "metabolic enhancer" Piracetem also suggest that this combination may be of some therapeutic utility. Research will continue and focus on the development of treatment and providing care and support to those with Alzheimer's and their families.

SIGNS AND SYMPTOMS OF DEMENTIA & MENTAL DISORDERS:

Emotional:	Physical:
Decrease in intellectual abilities	Loss of memory
Personality changes	Inability to visually
Depression – anxiety	discriminate
Lack of recall	weight increase
Communication difficulties	or loss
Delusions – hallucinations	Loss of motor ability
Irrational Suspiciousness	Body chemicals loss or

The treatment of mental disorders will depend on the diagnosis.

TIPS TO ASSIST A PERSON WITH DEMENTIA & MENTAL DISORDERS:

1. Doctor – Visit Regularly –Note Changes; treat medical problems promptly.

2. Routine – Maintain well-constructed, simple routines for daily activities; familiar persons, times of events, placement of possessions, etc.

3. Avoid stressful situations – These include unfamiliar persons, places and things.

4. Adaptation – Assist in adapting to a new environment; give reality orientation as necessary. Repeat directions specifically. Actualize a team care plan.

5. Never force or rush – Frequently, a person with dementia may not understand or cooperate with you. Do not push a subject to the point of agitation; try again later.

6. Communication – use both verbal and non-verbal communication skills. Maintain good eye contact; speak slowly with clearly understood words.

7. Agitation

   a). If the person says he/she is going to hit you. Get yourself and others out of the way and call for help.

   b). Find out why he/she is agitated and help him/her find a solution.

   c). Do not argue; do not correct harmless beliefs.

   d). Try to distract; do not over react.

   e). Do not embarrass him/her.

   f). Rummaging – give him/her a laundry basket or drawer to rummage in. Keep him/her busy with simple tasks. Make sure he/she isn't looking for something, like his/her teeth, the bathroom or towels. Let him/her have as many possessions as space will nearly and safely allow.

8. Wandering – make sure he/she has an ID bracelet, with phone number on it. Fence yards, within fire alarm, warning systems; be sure to keep a current picture of the consumer for identification purposes.

COMMUNICATION IN DEMENTIA

VERBAL

- Short words
- Simple sentences
- Identify yourself and call the person by name

SPEECH

- Speak slowly
- Say individual words clearly
- Lower the tone; raise the volume only for deafness, not because you do not get a response you understand
- Wait for a response
- Ask only one question at a time
- If you repeat a question repeat it exactly

NONVERBAL

- Every verbal communication is delivered with proper nonverbal gestures
- Maintain eye contact
- Move slowly
- If the person walks away while you are talking to him or her, do not try to stop him or her as your first move. Instead keep moving along in front of him and persevere.
- Listen actively. Ask for a repeat of the statement. Continue until resolution.
- Assume there is capability for insight.
- Compare notes on successes and failures.
- Treat the reaction with verbal/nonverbal techniques.
- If you have not really "gotten anywhere" in 5 minutes or less, you will probably do better to leave and either return in 5 minutes or have a colleague try.
- Finally, if you say you are going to do something, DO IT. If you forget, find the person and apologize. Assuming that the person has forgotten the episode insults both your intelligence and his/hers.
- If you need to stop a patient-patient interchange do it firmly and quickly. Get them out of each other's territory. Wait five minutes, then return and explain to each one why you acted as you did. Use factual explanations, not guilt induction.

LEVELS OF MENTAL DETERIORATION

LEVEL 1. MILD CONFUSION:

Notable decline in memory and concentration. Occasionally, gets disorientated as to place and time. Could get lost at times. Decrease in performance of activities of daily living. Difficulty in retaining information. Forgetful and misplaces belongings. Needs some supervision to maintain living standards.

LEVEL 2: EARLY DEMENTIA:

Unable to recall some family member's names. Difficulty counting backwards. Can no longer live alone – needs general supervision. Occasionally needs assistance with activities of daily living. Inability to recall recent some past experiences.

LEVEL 3: MIDDLE DEMENTIA:

Exhibits periods of anxiety and/or agitation. May forget child or spouse's name. Needs some assistance with activities of daily living. May need to be reminded to go to the bathroom and where the bathroom is. May show signs of insecurity and/or obsessive behavior. May lose thought during course of action. An example would be forgetting the process of eating during a meal. Needs over-all frequent supervision. May be living within a memory.

LEVEL 4: FINAL DEMENTIA

Diminished motor skills, may be unable to walk or feed self. Is incontinent. Speech is impaired, the majority of communication is lost. The brain is unable to tell the body what to do.

DELIRIUM

Symptoms of Delirium usually manifest themselves abruptly. They can be the sign of a serious underlying illness or disease which, if not diagnosed, can lead to death. A delirious person is described as confused and disoriented. He/she seems to have no short-term memory. Hallucinations and fears can occur. Often, the person will ramble or speak in disjointed sentences. If the symptoms are long-term, this person may need to be in a higher level of care.

SIGNS AND SYMPTOMS OF DELIRIUM:

Emotional:
Confusion
Illusions
Agitation
Short attention span
Fear

Physical:
Sleep disorders
Sweating
Rambling speech
Elevated blood pressure

Because the person may have an underlying illness or disease or can "freak out", it is essential to seek medical help if the symptoms abruptly surface.

SCHIZOPHRENIA

Schizophrenia varies in its severity from individual to individual. Those individuals are often referred to as crazy. They show odd behavior and talk nonsense. They may show odd behavior and talk nonsense. They may suffer with delusions and hallucinations. Schizophrenia generally can be controlled with medication and medical treatment.

Schizophrenia seems to worsen or improve in cycles known as relapse and remission, respectively. Sometimes, persons suffering from schizophrenia appear relatively normal. However, during a psychotic relapse, they cannot think logically and may lose all sense of who they are, what they are doing and where they are. Their thoughts are jumbled and chaotic.

Schizophrenia is considered one of the most baffling illnesses known. A person suffering from schizophrenia usually required treatment for the rest of his/her live. Depending on the extent of the disease, relative to that person, he/she may, or may not, be appropriate for consumer care.

INSOMNIA

Basically, we can divide insomnia into 3 sections:

1. Transient Insomnia (1 day to 1 week);
2. Short Term (1 to 3 weeks) and,
3. Chronic (3 weeks or longer)

When a consumer is having sleeping problems, be sure to document and keep a record, so pattern, if any, can be established. The doctor can best assess and advise how to assist a consumer when accurate information is provided. The types and times medication is given can affect sleeping. Has the consumer started any new medications? Has the consumer had stressful situations occurring in his/her life.
Is he/she having leg cramps or other pains? Are there environmental problems, such as light, temperature, noise, etc?

Sometimes, a consumer needs reassurance. A cup of herbal tea or warm milk with someone to talk over concerns and problems may be all he needs.

The following physical conditions can contribute to insomnia:

COPD (Chronic Obstructive Pulmonary Disease)
CHF (Congestive Heart Failure)
Anxiety
Asthma
Arthritis
Diuretics given at night
Headaches or Migraines
Epilepsy
Ulcers
Liver Failure
Diabetes
Kidney Failure
Infections
And many others.

EPILEPSY AND SEIZURE DISORDERS

When a person has "spells", "fits" or "convulsions", these signs may indicate a seizure. Most seizures are unpredictable. Some people have seizures from undetermined causes, others have been diagnosed with Epilepsy. Epilepsy is noted to cause a defect in the transmission of motor impulses in the brain. Seizure disorders and Epilepsy can usually be controlled by medication and the person can live a relatively normal life. However, it is essential that regular testing of the level of medication in the blood be done and evaluated periodically. Beverages containing alcohol should be avoided.

GRAND MAL SEIZURES

Sometimes a mood change or small contractions can indicate a possible seizure. The person usually falls, if not prevented from doing so. A loss of consciousness and convulsions occur, lasting from two to five minutes. Wild movements of the arms, legs and head transpire. After the person has regained consciousness, they will usually feel tired and want to sleep. Headaches and muscle soreness can occur.

PETIT MAL or ABSENCE SEIZURES

These types of seizures are usually characterized by the fluttering of the eye lids and small tremors of the head, arms and legs. The person will usually lose consciousness for 10 to 30 seconds. The seizures may occur frequently.

STATUS EPILEPTICUS or STATUS SEIZURES

These terms are used to describe rapid recurring seizures. The person doesn't usually regain consciousness between seizures. This is a serious condition and can be life threatening: CALL FOR IMMEDIATE MEDICAL ATTENTION.

OTHER TYPES OF SEIZURES include Facial Seizures, Psychomotor Seizures and Simple-Partial Seizures. The symptoms vary from facial twitching to mental confusion.

SIGNS AND SYMPTOMS OF SEIZURES:

MENTAL:	PHYSICAL:
Withdraws	Twitching
Staring Expression	Rigidity
Blackout	Convulsions

Confusion   Tremors
Hallucinations   Shaking
Loss of Consciousness   Jerking of extremities

HOW TO ASSIST: DO NOT PUT ANYTHING INTO THE MOUTH

1. If you notice any pre-seizure symptoms, get the person to sit or lie down.
2. If a person is undergoing a seizure, they should be lying down and turned on his/her side.
3. The head should be turned sideways to prevent saliva or tongue from clogging the throat.
4. Loosen clothing and remove any obstacles from the surrounding area.
5. Keep him from hurting himself, but allow freedom of movement.

RECORDS TIME, DURATION AND SITUATION. ALWAYS MAKE SURE HE/SHE SEES THE ATTENDING PHYSICIAN REGULARLY.

PARKINSON'S DISEASE

Parkinson's disease is a group of degenerative neurological disorders, generally characterized by uncontrolled movements of the body's extremities; i.e. shaking, tremors, rigidity of the muscles can occur. The person may show signs of sluggishness or shuffling. It occurs in a small percent of the elderly affecting both men and women.

Science has shown it is the result of the degeneration of certain types of brain cells. The production and storage of a type of neurotransmitter called Dopamine is depleted. There is also indications of Acetylcholine concentrations, another type of neurotransmitter. Anticholinergic or Dopamine medications may be used specifically or together as a treatment.

The onset of Parkinson's is usually gradual, developing over many years. Changes in posture, stiffness or shaking of the hands, weakness and slowness of movement are among some of the many symptoms. Treatment varies from each individual. Physical therapy and the use of environmental aids can often help. Support from family, friends and the care givers is fundamental. As in most types of chronic illnesses, anxiety and depression can develop. The combined treatment of medications, therapy, and supportive loving care can help the person function almost for many years.

PLEASE NOTE: Parkinson's type symptoms can result from medications used in treating mental illness and other diseases. Arteriosclerosis and other disorders may also cause Parkinson's Disease.

SIGNS AND SYMPTOMS OF PARKINSON'S

Fatigue or Weakness   Lack of Affect (facial expression)
Shaking or Tremors   Limping or Shuffling
Stoop or Poor posture Slowed Speech
Difficult Swallowing Muscular Rigidity
Drooling

TIPS TO ASSIST:

1. Regular checkup by the attending physician

2. Encourage a moderate exercise program (Range of motion exercises help keep limbs limber)

3. Let the consumer practice reading out loud if he is having difficulty with slow or slurred speech

4. Remind person who shuffles to pick up his/her feet.

5. Remind person who is stooping or slouching to correct posture.

6. Provide easy to-get-up from chairs, beds and toilets

VISION PROBLEMS

Many older persons suffer from vision problems. The most common type of problems include cataracts, glaucoma, macular degeneration, and diabetic retinopathy.

MUCULAR DEGENERATION

The macula is the small pigmented area of the retina. Degeneration of the macula is the leading cause of severe vision loss among the elderly. The macula controls the fine vision. The deterioration leads to blurring and/or loss in central vision.

Signs and Symptoms of Macular Degeneration:

1. Vision will be fuzzy.
2. Straight lines will appear wavy or doubled.
3. Letters will appear jumbled.

If the degeneration has not caused a total loss of vision, many times a magnifying glass can still be utilized.

Policies and Procedures

MEDICATIONS

MEDICATIONS HOW, WHY, WHEN, AND WHERE.

The regulations pertaining to medications in Title 22 are should be read and frequently reviewed by Administrator and staff. It is very important to prepare a proper medication disbursement system.

OUR SYSTEM

The medications storage and preparation site is placed in the area near hand washing facilities. Anyone assisting with medications should wash his/her hands first. There will be a telephone located close to the medication storage site to relay information to Physician, pharmacist, etc... Every medication must be logged in on LIC form # 622, in the record which is to be kept for each resident.

The resident's records must be kept or inaccessible. The records are confidential. A separate box, basket or section, with each resident's full name and room number on it, should be kept to retain his/her prescriptions and over-the-counter medications. A centralized Med Storage will be locked at all times.

ASSISTING WITH MEDICATIONS

After washing hands, staff must wear gloves and it is a good idea to use the lid of the bottle to pour the pills into and then the directed amount into the pill cup or placed in a cup separate from a drinking cup for the consumer to take. Paper and plastic pill cups can be purchased from some local pharmacy or a medical suppliers.

BUBBLE/BLISTER PACKS

The most efficient and controllable medication system is the bubble or blister pack, with a thirty day supply on a single card. This card can be initialed by the staff person each time the drug is punched out, certifying that the resident was seen taking medication.

RESIDENT'S REFUSAL OF A MEDICATION

The staff trained to provide medication is responsible for making sure that the resident is properly taking his/her medications. If a resident refuses a medication, which he/she can do, you must document it in their record and notify the physician. The physician may choose to discontinue the medication. But if the doctor feels that discontinuance is detrimental to the resident's health, he should help the Home in getting the resident transferred to a more appropriate facility.

Factual Scenario:

A facility once had a resident, "Mr. Smith," who was found to be spitting his thyroid pills in the toilet. He was informed that the "house rules" stated that all residents must take their medicines as Doctor prescribed and that any violation of the "house rules" were grounds for eviction. Mr. Smith transferred to another facility. Fortunately, he did. If he had died, our home would most likely have been held responsible for his death by CCL.

STORAGE OF MEDICATIONS

All medications will be stored in a locked and centrally located storage cabinet. PRN "as needed" MEDICATIONS

PRN comes from the Latin (pro re nata) "as the need arises". In our home it should mean "as requested by the resident". Prior to admission, or prior to the start of a new medication, you must obtain a written statement from the attending
BUBBLE/BLISTER PACKS

The most efficient and controllable medication system is the bubble or blister pack, with a thirty day supply on a single card. This card can be initialed by the staff person each time the drug is punched out, certifying that the resident was seen taking medication.

RESIDENT'S REFUSAL OF A MEDICATION

The staff trained to provide medication is responsible for making sure that the resident is properly taking his/her medications. If a resident refuses a medication, which he/she can do, you must document it in their record and notify the physician. The physician may choose to discontinue the medication. But if the doctor feels that discontinuance is detrimental to the resident's health, he should help the Home in getting the resident transferred to a more appropriate facility.

Factual Scenario:

A facility once had a resident, "Mr. Smith," who was found to be spitting his thyroid pills in the toilet. He was informed that the "house rules" stated that all residents must take their medicines as Doctor prescribed and that any violation of the "house rules" were grounds for eviction. Mr. Smith transferred to another facility. Fortunately, he did. If he had died, our home would most likely have been held responsible for his death by CCL.

STORAGE OF MEDICATIONS

All medications will be stored in a locked and centrally located storage cabinet. PRN "as needed" MEDICATIONS

PRN comes from the Latin (pro re nata) "as the need arises". In our home it should mean "as requested by the resident". Prior to admission, or prior to the start of a new medication, you must obtain a written statement from the attending physician that the resident is mentally capable of determining his/her need for that PRN medicine. When a resident requests a PRN medication, staff needs to document the amount taken, date, time, result and they should sign or initial it. This will eliminate the chance of overdose and provide an accurate record of usage. When a resident can't determine his/her own need for a PRN medication, the Doctor must be contacted and his/her permission granted before that medication is given. If the Doctor gives specific instructions as to dose, date and time, then it is no longer considered a PRN medication. Only the Doctor, not family or friends can give you permission to give a PRN medication when the resident is unable to determine this for himself/herself. Always document Doctor instructions; put the date, time and sign or initial it. Then you need to document the result on the resident's record.

Residents should be cautious when using OTC's if they have any of the following conditions:

- Arthritis
- Diabetes
- Glaucoma
- Heart disease
- High blood pressure
- Kidney disease
- Nervous condition
- Sleep problems

The most common medical conditions affected by OTC's are:

- Gout
- Prostate problems
- Ulcers

Questions which should be asked of the doctor or pharmacist regarding use of OTC's:

1. Can the resident take this OTC?

2. Will it be effective?

3. How long can he/she take it?

4. Will it interact adversely with other medications the resident is taking?

TIPS TO REMEMBER

1. Always keep records of OTC's and frequency of use.

2. Encourage resident to drink 8 ounces of water when taking medication.

3. Antacids and laxatives are best taken 2 hours before or after taking other medications.

4. Remember to read "Warnings and Precautions"

MEDICATION POLICY

An individual medication log for each resident shall be maintained. Information shall include the following:

Resident's name

Physician's name prescribing the medicine

Name of medicine, date prescription is filled

Direction, strength and amount

Pharmacy name & phone number

RX number, expiration date & number of refills

This log will be kept in the resident's records. All medicine, including over-the-counter medicine, shall be kept under lock and key, either in the locked cabinet or at the bedside in a locked box.

The Shift Supervisor shall give assistance with prescribed medications which are self-administered in accordance with the physician's instructions. We are not licensed for, and will not give, any injections or medication the resident cannot self-administer, unless we have employed an Appropriately Skilled Professional (ASP) who is licensed or certified to perform these duties in the State of California and it is within the governing regulation for a Residential Care Facility.

RESTRICTIONS ON "SETTING UP" AND "DRAWING UP" INJECTABLES

Insulin and other injectable medications shall be kept in their original containers until the prescribed single dose is measured into a syringe for immediate injection. Dosages of insulin and other injectable medications shall not be prepared or "set up" in advance by filling one or more syringes with the prescribed dose and storing medication in the syringe until needed. The prohibition of advance set-up does not apply to medications that are packaged by a pharmacist or a manufacturer in pre-measured doses in individual syringes.

Only the resident or certified medical professionals are permitted to mix injectable medication prescribed for the resident or to fill the syringe with the prescribed dose ("draw up" the medication). The medical professionals permitted to administer medications include only physicians, registered nurses and licensed vocational nurses.

HOUSE SUPPLIES

OVER-THE-COUNTER MEDS

(Before assisting the residents with these kinds of medications, get doctor's approval)
Acetaminophen (Tylenol, etc.)
Milk of Magnesia
Fleet Enema(for residents' self-use or ASP)
Metamucil

Anusol suppositories (for residents' self-use or ASP)
ExLax
Bisacodyl
Ecotrin, aspirin
Rolaids
Tums
Mineral Oil
Castor Oil
Glycerin suppositories (for residents' self-use or ASP)
Listerine
Boric Acid
Cough drops
Guituss-Dm, Robitussin (coughs and colds medicine)
NOTE: REMEMBER TO CHECK EXPIRATION DATES

FIRST AID SUPPLIES

Bandages, Plastic Strip 2" x 4 ½" (Band-Aid, etc.)
Bandages, Elastic Knee & Elbow 2" x 4" (Ace)
Bandages, Plastic, various shapes and sizes (Band-Aid, etc.)
Telfa non-stick pads 3" x 4"
Adhesive Tape, Water –proof ½" and 1" rolls
Cotton Balls
Alcohol Swabs
Cloth Tape
Butterfly Closures
Steri-strips
Tegaderm
Duo-Derm
Biolex
Disposable gloves
Providine solution
Hydrogen Peroxide
A & D ointment
Vaseline Intensive Care Lotion
Calmine lotion
Campho Phenique
Ben Gay
Muscle Rrub
Rubbing Alcohol
KY Jelly

PLANNED ACTIVITIES OF COMMUNITY RESOURCES:

Daily activities are highly structured and require constant supervision. Activities are planned by residents and supervisor and are integral to, not separate from, resident's treatment. More resident's level of mental, social, psychological capacity shall an important factor in preparation of residents activities. Our goal will be to help residents with acceptable decision making, interaction in community activities, as well as participation in planned program activities.

Examples of planned outdoor activities include the following: Sports and athletics, use of exercise equipment, basketball, volleyball, ping-pong, gymnastics, aerobics and dance, movies, stage productions, museums, camping, beach outings, skating, picnics, amusement parks, T.V. shows. Indoor activities include crafts, word and board games, sewing, cooking, reading, art projects, computer games, etc. In addition to the planned activities in the facility, residents participate in planned activities outside the facility. Each month a cultural activity to broaden their knowledge of the world around them.

The frequency of activities which are planned for the residents take into account the levels of functioning. Opportunities for solitary, parallel, associative and cooperative activities are included in the program. Examples of planned solitary activities include the following: cards, games, skateboarding, puzzles, and crafts, reading, listening to tapes, jazzercize, etc. examples of planned parallel activities include watching movies, singing, walking, biking, playing games, ping-pong, baking cookies, art projects, dance, and singing.

Community resources used by AngelCare Home include: libraries, local churches, Claremont Youth Activity Center, parks and recreation, YMCA, Cal Poly University, Local Colleges, Grisworld's Community Theater, Los Angeles County Fair, The Grove Theater (stage plays), Chino Community Theater, San Bernardino County Independent Living Program, local businesses, Women's Foundation, County Community Foundation (Grants to finance activities), Title 1 L.A. Co. Office of Education – Division of Alternative Education. The administrator or designee will evaluate and approve all activities prior to the event.

The residents are encouraged to participate in recreational activities. We encourage participation by having various exercise equipment readily available at home, these include, basketball courts, volleyball nets and balls, cardio-glide riders, stationary bikes, hand weights, slant boards, jazzercise and other exercise and dance to music videos. Our home shall have bikes and helmets so they can tour the neighborhood accompanied by a staff member. Hiking in the nearby hills with staff, jogging around the school running track, roller skating sessions and bowling outings are all popular activities with the residents. We also plan weekly picnics at nearby parks with the residents providing basketball or volleyball teams to compete in friendly playoffs.

The residents will be provided education programs available through the local schools, day programs, adult schools, or colleges. These programs may include attendance at the regular school classes or an individually designed program, opportunity classes, extension classes.

Recognizing the critical importance of the educational experience in the residents overall treatment, the treatment team regards the Regional Center as a cooperative partner in providing services to residents. Because of the nature of our home clientele, both the individual resident and school personnel require substantial support in developing and maintaining a successful educational experience for these adult residents. Day program/school attendance is closely monitored by facility managers.

DISCHARGE/REMOVAL

The home operates a long term program with residency expected to be 12 months or longer. Planned terminations are of three types: a.) reunification with family of origin, b) placement or transfer to a less structured treatment program   c) others.

EMERGENCY DISCHARGE:

Unplanned terminations are generally the result of inability or non-participation in policies and procedures due to health issues. However a resident's behavior or failure to comply with the program, may result in a request from the home to have a resident removed. In an attempt to prevent moving residents, a case conference with case worker will be requested; however, if residents behavior is disruptive to other residents placement termination will be requested.

RUNAWAYS:

In the event of an AWOL, the following actions are taken. The staff person on duty will notify police if the resident does not call or appear within 1 hour after the designated time to return. The referring agency social worker/probation offices, consultant and licensing will be notified within 24 hours. If AWOL occurs on a weekend, they will be notified on the first working day after the AWOL. Representatives will be notified when the Home will hold the resident's place for up to 5 days. In the event the resident returns, the therapist will interview the resident to determine an appropriate course of action. Because the program is designed to work with chronic placement failures, which include runaways, the potential for AWOL behavior is minimized by the treatment team providing appropriate intervention. The program will generally be willing to hold a residents place if some progress toward treatment goals is being made.

CLOTHING: INITIAL CLOTHING:

Upon admission, a residents clothing is inventoried by the case worker and the staff. If a new resident does not have adequate clothing as required by the Regional Center, an emergency purchase order to cover the cost will be requested from the placing agency and additional clothing will be purchased. The administration approves purchase orders and issues funds for the clothing. Client's will be taken shopping and their choices of clothing must be approved for appropriateness, affordability, durability and clothing requirements, by the accompanying staff.

PROCEDURES FOR SAFEGUARDING CLOTHING AND PERSONAL PROPERTY:

In the event of a planned termination, the staff will assist a resident in packing her belongings, ensuring that she leaves with her and only her clothing and personal property. In regard to unplanned terminations, resident's clothing and personal belongings are locked in secure storage in the facility. The consumer's representative will be notified to pick up client's personal belongings. All personal clothing and property will be held for thirty (30) days, at which time all times will be donated to a charitable organization.

RELIGIOUS SERVICES:

Residents who need supervision and who wish to attend religious services need to notify manager by 4:00 pm on Friday, in order for to arrange for supervision. Transportation to a church temple, or other religious facility of the residents choice within the community will be provided by the Home vans and personnel. Volunteers whose licenses and insurance are on file with AngelCare Home may be utilized to accompany residents to these services.

Residents who are able to be out for a limited time without supervision, will be transported by the Home to the religious facility of their choice and picked up after the conclusion of services. For residents who choose not of attend church, alternative activities will be provided. These house activities will include board and computer games, videos, exercise equipment and books and magazines. Supervision is always provided!

INTERNAL COMMUNICATION RECORD:

Staff will maintain individual behavioral records on each records on each resident. All staff are responsible for recording daily behaviors and the social milieu of the day. Incoming staff review log notes for relative information. All records are reviewed weekly by the facility manager. The administrator or designee will review a sampling of the log notes to insure appropriate records are maintained. Logs are maintained that reflect records of home visits and unsupervised time in the community. See attachment – Daily Log Notes. Social workers review log notes Monday thru Friday on a daily basis to update their knowledge of their residents. The Administrator or her designee review samples of log notes twice monthly.

All medical records will be maintained in the medical log with results of the appointments. A resident on a family pass be signed out by the person authorized to pick her up for the visit. The phone number and address of the family must on record. The person authorized to return the resident must sign her back into the facility. (See attachment- Sign in Sheet)

Exhibit Three: : Sample Business Plan

ANGELCARE COMPANY, INC.

A Business Plan to Establish a Vocational and Recreation Center in the Inland Empire Area.

AngelCare Day Program

A Business Plan

*Research made exclusively for ANGEL CARE Company, Inc.
By: HealthCare Training and Staffing Services ®.
September 01, 2004*

Table of Contents

1. EXECUTIVE SUMMARY: 333
2. OBJECTIVES 334
    1.1 HIGHLIGHTS: Graph
3. MISSION 335
4. COMPANY SUMMARY 335
5. COMPANY OWNERSHIP 336
6. START-UP SUMMARY 337
7. SERVICES 338
    6.0 START UP GRAPH
    Table 6.1 Start-Up Cost
8. MARKET ANALYSIS 341
9. MARKET SEGMENTATION 342
    Graph 9.1: Area Segmentation
    Table 9.1: Market Analysis
10. TARGET MARKET SEGMENT STRATEGY 342
11. SERVICE BUSINESS ANALYSIS 343
12. COMPETITION AND BUYING PATTERNS 343
13. STRATEGY AND IMPLEMENTATION 345
14. COMPETITIVE EDGE 346
15. SALES FORECAST 347
    GRAPH: SALES MONTHLY
    Table 3.0 Sales Forecast
16. MILESTONES 348
    Table 16.0 Milestones
17. MANAGEMENT SUMMARY 348
18. PERSONNEL PLAN 349
    Table 18.1 Personnel Plan
19. FINANCIAL PLAN 349
20. IMPORTANT ASSUMPTIONS 350
    Table: 20.1 General Assumptions
21. BREAK EVEN ANALYSIS 350
    Graph: 21.1 Break Even Analysis

Table: 21.1 Break Even Analysis
22. PROJECTED PROFIT AND LOSS 351
Table 22.1 Profit and Loss Statement
23. PROJECTED CASH FLOW 351
Graph: 23.1: Cash Flow
24. PROJECTED BALANCE SHEET 352
Table 24.1: Balance Sheet
USEFUL CONTACT INFORMATION 353
Other Resources 356
Glossary of words 357

1. EXECUTIVE SUMMARY:

ANGELCARE Day Program for Seniors and Adults is a service oriented type of business that will cater to the needs of individuals with disabilities specifically those living within the counties of San Bernardino and Riverside. The business is established as a result of an overwhelming demand for a unique type of an adult day care (ADC) program that will provide vocational and habilitation training, mentorship and job placements, behavioral modification and therapy all under one service objective. The center shall be used for community based as well as center based program of activities to serve the needs of a wide range of disabled and aging consumers mostly from Inland Regional Center and from the Department of Aging.

The individualized service plan shall take into consideration the specific consumer needs and services, their functional ability, the consumers challenges, their behaviors and their ability to retain and respond to given task.

It is a unique concept-program in a sense that the goal is to provide the service to the consumers in a recreational and leisurely manner and that the adult day care center program shall be used for a dual purpose wherein during the day time, the center shall be used as a day care center for adults and seniors, while after work hours, such as Fridays and Saturdays, the center shall be used as an activity center or recreational hall similar to a " sports bar " or a dance studio where consumers spend a couple of hours socializing with their friends and significant others to enhance and develop their social and recreational skills.

As of this time, there is no existing program like it and this organization would like to introduce this break through concept to be able to accommodate the expanding needs of our consumers and to provide a wide variety of options for our consumers where they will be able to apply the social and recreational skills they learn from their schools, day programs and at home.

1.1 HIGHLIGHTS: Graph

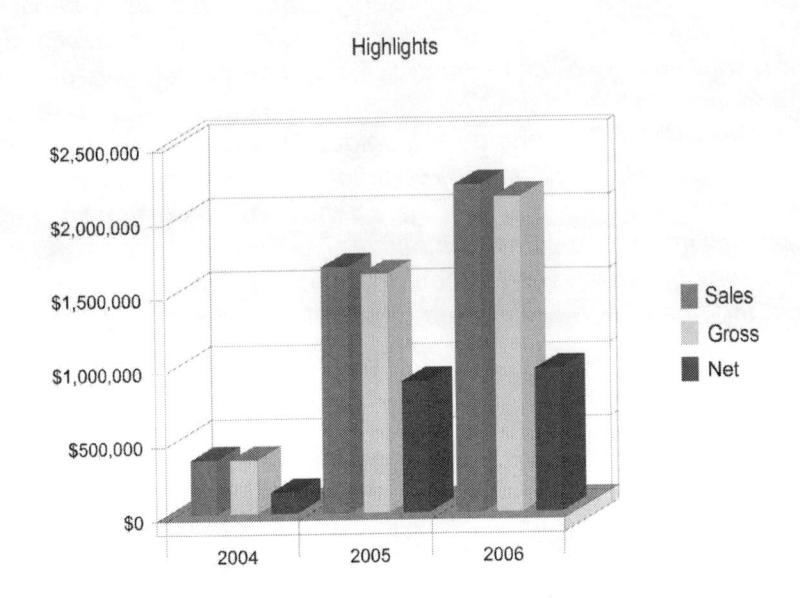

Highlights

[Bar chart showing Sales, Gross, and Net for years 2004, 2005, and 2006, with values ranging from $0 to $2,500,000]

2. OBJECTIVES

The Objectives of our business are as follows:

1. To provide a unique multi-purpose adult day care center that shall serve primarily as a center-based program with community-based components offering habilitation, therapeutic environment with behavioral components, mentoring and employment as well as a dual purpose day program cum leisure and recreation center.

2. To maintain our projected start-up cost of approximately $45,000.00 (or a total cash reserve of $ 100,000.00 to be able to show our financial capability with the bank as well as Community Care Licensing in launching this business.

3. Our Projected Sales of $363,000 by fiscal year 2004 and exceeding $2 Million Dollars by fiscal years 2005-2006.

4. It is our goal to exceed our gross margin higher than 45% on our second year and reach our maximum projections by year 2005.

5. A net income of more than 30% of sales by the third year and reach our net profit / sales by 53% by the year 2005.

3. MISSION

Angel Care Day Program for Seniors and Adults offers a unique adult day care programming (ADC) combined as a recreation center will provide center-based as well as community-based day program activities as a true alternative to currently existing adult day care centers.

A true alternative in a sense that it will offer day programming activities focused on the individual's needs and services, disabilities, potentials, learning curve, behaviors and most of all to enhance the consumers' social and recreational skills. Care Day Program offers a wide variety of activities, behavior modification components, therapy, mentorship and job placements; and at the same time could be used as a recreational center where consumers socialize, watch a movie, dance or sing to a Karaoke night and consume food and non-alcoholic beverages including freshly made juices of their choice.

4. COMPANY SUMMARY

ANGELCARE COMPANY, INC. is a new company that will establish an adult day care center in the Inland Empire area and it shall be called ANGELCARE Day Program. This company is proud to be the first to introduce a revolutionary approach in adult day care programming where it shall rise above the standards of your average day program as it will introduce to the public a unique approach to activities, therapy, community integration, socialization and most of all, it shall be the center for two important activities for our consumers: day programming and recreation center where they will be able to enjoy encounters and interactions with friends in a club/bar setting where they can watch movies, sing-along with a friend and enjoy a non-alcoholic beverage or just simply to spend time in a place similar to a dance club.

ANGELCARE Company, Inc. will provide the best quality day programming activities equipped with the latest techniques that are unorthodox in approach. This will be totally different and revolutionary in approach compared to your typical day program in a sense that the program design is focused mainly on the individual client's needs and not as a group setting.

The company may probably be new per se but it shall be composed of experienced health care professional staff and consultants from the fields of psychiatry, medicine, behavior analysis, occupational and physical therapy and mental-physics.

The company shall start conservatively with one main office which shall be located within the Inland Empire area to eventually grow depending on the ongoing demand for the service.

5. COMPANY OWNERSHIP

ANGELCARE Day Program will be established by ANGELCARE Company, Inc., as part of its initial project in the health care field. Care company, Inc. is owned and operated by its board of directors and members as principal investors and principal operators. The initial business address of the company shall be located at 123 A Street, B City, Ca. 123456. Telephone (800) 456-7890. The initial board of directors are as follows:

      Mr. Joe Sample, President
      Ms. Mary Sample, V-President
      Mrs. Onlee Sample, Secretary
      Mrs. Onlee sample, Treasurer
      Mr. Onlee Wan Sample, Chief Finance Officer

The Care Day Program for seniors and Adults shall be managed and administered by Mr. Onlee Sample, Regional Administrator, Mrs. Onlee Wan Sample, Director for Operations and Assistant

Administrator. The Program Director position is currently under negotiation available pending this study and shall be filled prior to the facility acquiring a license to operate as day care center which shall be granted by Community Care Licensing and Inland Regional Center. Said position is currently being offered to an individual with at least three years of day program management and operations and preferably with a masters degree in similar field.

6. START-UP SUMMARY

The start up cost for Care Day Program for Seniors and Adults with Developmental Disabilities is approximately $45,139.00. to pay for our initial fixed and variable costs as well as to meet our expenses in constructing and developing our ideal day program site. We project based on conservative estimates that approximately $26,899.00 will be spent effectively for our expenses on the application process, office equipment and supplies, day program equipment and supplies and renovation of the program site. Part of our initial cost shall include expenses for the following:

> Incorporation expenses
> Research and development
> Certification classes
> Consultancy
> Legal cost
> Office supplies
> Computers
> Site improvement
> Purchase of facility equipment and educational tools
> and other expenses associated
> with opening its first office.
> Miscellaneous expenses

During our initial operation, we will be utilizing our investors funds to register our company with the Secretary of State of California. After registration, we will be purchasing office equipment and supplies, facility equipment and tables, chairs and cabinets, educational materials to decorate our site. Most of the furniture will be purchased from an auction sale and shall be in very good condition which will be integrated with our facility design patterned after functional and practical purposes.

Our estimated total asset is at $ 45,000.00 and our total start up requirement is $99,859.00 to cover our initial operating cost starting in January 2004 wherein such funds will be used to cover three months of operations. We project that by the month of May 2004, we shall expect our first batch of clients after three months of marketing our company with residential care facilities located within our target area. By the months of May and June 2004, we will be expecting shortage in operating capital due to our operating cost which is starting to consume approximately 75% of our accumulated funds, therefore, it will be a practical and imperative approach to infuse additional $10,000 during the month of May and an additional $10,000 by June. In order to avoid this additional capital infusion, the investors as well as the Regional Director and Assistant Program Director shall be earning a salary credit which will be refunded by the early months of 2005 when revenues are starting to climb at a comfortable level.

6.0 START UP GRAPH

Table 6.1 Start-Up Cost

7. SERVICES

ANGELCARE Day Program also known as CARE shall offer the highest quality in day programming activities to be able to capture at a minimum the 10% of the existing market. The objective of the company is to be able to attract existing day program clients including future clients residing in care facilities, apartments, private homes, retirement homes, assisted living as well those individuals living independently at home on their own. The goal is to offer a different but unique programming approach to habilitation, social and recreational activities focused on the individualized needs of the consumers. The program is both center based as well as community based depending on the clients' needs and services, behavior and developmental capacity. The program believes in the approach... " that no consumer shall be at home for any reason other than medical, dental and self choice". Contrary to what most day program do, Care Day program shall attempt to accommodate every consumers' need regardless of the issue whether it be behavioral, emotional or psychological. A program plan shall be developed individually to accommodate their needs and to keep them in the day program as possible and to learn and participate in the daily activities whether it be in the community or at the center.

Angel Care Day program shall offer the following component services with emphasis on the clients' choice, rights and self-advocacy:

A.   Community Based Day Program

Focused primarily on providing the consumers with creative and functional-educational activities, to learn the much needed skills and provide an all natural, unrestricted environment of free choice for learning and personal growth. In order to achieve this, the company shall exert its best effort and resources in maximizing the utilization of community resources, funding and support from other entities, public agencies as well as private entities. The day program activities shall consist of 5.5 hours of community involvement and participation in the community such as cleaning churches, parks and recreation, movie theaters etc... This is the individual's way of learning the basic skills similar to a job or volunteer program.

B. Center Based Day Program

1. **Work Training Program** by providing a wide variety of vocational training sites within the community. These work sites shall be developed by Angel Care Vocational Services and Recreation Center where consumers will be given the opportunity to learn the much needed skills relative to their quest in gaining employment. The program requires full supervision with sufficient client to staff ratio conducive towards the attainment of the consumers' goals.

2. **Habilitation Program.** Focused on functional skills and needs of the consumers, the program shall provide supervised training

on the use of home equipments, cooking utensils etc.. The goal is to familiarize the consumers with the life of self-reliance and independence by learning to cook, food preparation, housekeeping and home maintenance.

3. **Develop personal, social, recreational, tactile and other related skills.** The program will promote the individualized development of personal self-care, feeding, occupational and recreational skills by providing age appropriate equipment, tools of learning and resources needed to enhance the individuals personal capacity. The consumers will be treated to a monthly trip to special places of interest such as museums, parks, camping trips, trips to the casino and other interesting places that consumers prefer in order to enhance their social and recreational skills.

4. **Independent Living Program.** To promote self-reliance and confidence to the consumers, the program will provide supervised training staff to assists the consumers in community participation and to enhance their personal experiences within the community by facilitating positive interaction with others, within the community and of course their own home environment or community. The program shall provide training, assistance and support in various areas of community integration. Part of the clients' learning expectations include safety at home and in public, parenting skills, mobility training and assistance in accessing community resources.

5. **On the job Training and Supervision, Job Placements.** Providing career counseling, planning and mentoring. Angel Care shall secure job placements through Dept. of Rehabilitation assistance, etc.

6. **Physical, recreational, occupational and emotional therapy.** Providing consumers with activities that will enhance their physical, recreational and emotional needs such as morning exercises, walks to the parks, aromatherapy, interactive-music, computer familiarization, a big screen television where weekly special movies in a theater like setting will be provided, Friday and Saturday dance nights and Karaoke nights, every month particularly on a last Friday of the month, there shall be talent shows and consumer participation. The consumers will be taken to a public land where they will participate in community participation where they will go out into

the community to do volunteer clean ups of forest, beaches, parks and recreation to show their support to the community programs.

7. **Behavior modification.** In order to keep the consumers active in the day center, they will be provided with a 1:1 or a 3:1 staff to consumer ratio in the event that they become non-conforming to the program, when behavior becomes an issue, instead of sending the consumer (s) home, a behaviorist will be available to draw up a program plan to address their individual behavior which will be executed by a staff familiar with the consumer in particular.

8. **Transition planning.** Proving the consumer(s) with a program to help them learn the basics of independent living such as lessons in cooking, gardening, safety, self-reliance in case of an emergency, food and material purchasing, budgeting, money management, housekeeping, job search and interviewing, etc...

9. **Transportation.** The program shall include availability of transportation through staff transport, a non-mobile/mobile van/ bus to transport the consumers to and from their homes and other locations relative to their needs and services.

The program shall initially start with a community based activities to enhance social and community integration which eventually transition to center based activities or vice versa.

8. MARKET ANALYSIS

ANGELCARE Day Program will focus on providing the best quality adult day care programming to individuals with disabilities including seniors living privately at home as well as those living in residential care facilities. The adult day care center shall be located in the City of Sample, California between the 10 freeway and the 15 freeway to be able service the needs of the local residents as well as those in neighboring cities where there is an urgent need for an adult day care center. Our target market area shall be consumers of Regional Center and Private individuals residing within the cities of Claremont, Upland, Chino, Pomona, Diamond Bar, Alta Loma, Rancho Cucamonga, San Dimas, Montclair, Corona, Fontana,

Colton, Apple Valley, Temecula, Palmdale, Victorville and other neighboring cities. All these cities are divided into areas one, two, three and four respectively

Our most potential group of clientele are those coming from local residential care facilities within the 25-30 mile radius from our adult day care enter where there is an urgent need for it due to the lack of availability of local resources such as an adult day care as well as the lack of good quality programming activities.

9. MARKET SEGMENTATION

1. The largest group of clienteles are coming from the residential care homes which has an average of six residents per household. All these consumers are coming from the both agencies of San Gabriel-Pomona and Inland Empire areas specifically from Pomona, Diamond Bar, Chino, Chino hills, Claremont, Montclair, Upland, Ontario, Fontana, Rancho Cucamonga, Rialto, Temecula and Perris areas.

2. The second largest group of possible clients shall be coming from Rialto, Corona, Riverside and Norco areas.

3. And the third group of clients are from the upper desert region including Palmdale, Lancaster, Victorville, Apple Valley and neighboring dessert cities where there is one to none available day programs.

Graph 9.1: Area Segmentation

Table 9.1: Market Analysis

10. TARGET MARKET SEGMENT STRATEGY

The strategy behind our market segmentation is listening to the needs of the community, the consumers and most of all the request of Inland Regional Center, Dept. of Aging, Dept. of Health Services and other entities by regularly updating our resources, program and services to meet the evolving demand for our services on as needed and or as necessary as possible. We will maintain flexibility, practicality and most of all adaptability to the consumers' ever changing needs.

Another focal point for our reference shall be the variety of services we will provide to our consumers, the quality of our services which follows the highest standard of care and supervision, our consistency in our staffing ratio to consumers which is an average of 1:4 to maintain high quality standard as well as continuous training of our staff and most of all our focus on safety and cleanliness at the work place to make it conducive for learning and a good working environment for our consumers as well as our staff.

11. SERVICE BUSINESS ANALYSIS

The adult day care business is very popular education and vocational alternative among residential care facility for adults and seniors with disabilities. Due to the consumers varied disabilities, they will have a difficult time coping with standards of regular schools of learning, thus a special school of learning was created and they could come in different varieties and one of these special educational schools may come ideally as a day care center also known popularly called as "day program". This concept was introduced to be able meet the growing demand for special education schools or training centers to meet the needs of more than 18,000 consumers residing within the counties of San Bernardino and Riverside Counties. For this reason, we would like to participate by capturing at least 10% of the existing client market base.

12. COMPETITION AND BUYING PATTERNS

The key element in adult day care business is the excellent relationship between the day program, the care-provider as well as Regional Center case managers who arranges the purchasing of these much needed services. The determining factors in choosing day program for the consumers are as follows:

> Quality of care and supervision
>
> Safety and cleanliness of the site.
>
> Staffing based on the program offered which requires courtesy, respect, freedom from abuse and neglect, experience and education maintained by the staff in general.
>
> Program variety, practical application and consistency.
>
> Consistency in programming and follow-up on consumer's progress and development.
>
> How the consumers will be able to learn and enjoy his activities that address their needs and services.

It is however of utmost importance for the consumer to be able to enjoy the activities offered at the day program as well as the consumers' benefits of being there on a daily basis such as the approach to learning, the type of activities offered, the quality of service and experience and professionalism among counselors and support staff at the day program.

The average price for the programming services is at $ 65.00 /day per consumer.

THE COMPETITION:

1. Sample Day program
2. Wan sample day program
3. LOPARC-
4. POARC
5. FOPARC
6. MOPARC

Despite of the intimidating number of available day care centers as competitors in our target area, the population has grown considerably in the past five years that the demand is undeniably still unmet up to this date. The outgrown and still growing number of residential care facilities in our area, the demand is outnumbers the available resources that is why we are confident that our program will always be in demand. Our program is so unique in its purpose and scope of services that other care-providers will be willing to try our services and experience the enormous differences in concept, programming, variety and practicality. With our best selling leisure center our consumers will be given the opportunity to interact with others, develop and apply their learned social skills apply it in an environment similar to that of a day club or a sports bar.

13. STRATEGY AND IMPLEMENTATION

AngelCare Day Program will focus on various geographical markets namely:

1. **Area One:** Diamond Bar, Chino, Chino Hills, Claremont, Montclair,

2. **Area Two:** Upland, Rancho Cucamonga, Ontario, Etiwanda,

3. **Area Three:** Fontana, Rialto, Corona, Temecula, Perris,

4. **Area Four:** Victorville, Apple Valley and other neighboring Upper Dessert areas where day program is deeply necessary.

Our target clients are coming from different residential care facilities for adults and seniors, community care facilities levels 1-4 and private families living within the abovementioned geographical areas.

The company's competitive edge is the fact that we offer a very unique program, one that is revolutionary in approach and totally in demand. We are not your average day program that offers more than the norm. Our day care center starts it operation initially as community based program were consumers will be provided transportation to and from the center where designated staff will join them and will be taken to the community where they will be able to learn the skills needed to contribute to the society such as community clean ups, job search, community volunteer programs, habilitation, behavior modification, social integration, etc... As soon as the facility site is available, we will integrate center based programming to our consumers whom we will alternate depending on their assessment, behavior and evaluation.

One of our unique characteristic is that we are capable of accommodating consumers who needs behavior modification, 1:1 programming, counseling, individualized therapy sessions.

With our target location which is strategically suitable for consumers living within the 20-30 mile radius, transportation will not be an issue specifically in relation to daily programming, emergencies, social integration, resource accessibility and best of all our close proximity to the three major freeways where 90% of our consumers will be coming from different cities proximately located to the day care center.

14. COMPETITIVE EDGE

Our best selling point is our unique program statement where we will be able to cater to the needs of both adults and seniors with low functioning up to those with high functioning capabilities, therefore our services will encompass a wide variety of community as well as center based activities that will benefit a wide array of consumer needs. We will be providing behavior modification programming for difficult to deal with consumers and provide them with activities appropriate to their needs. The revolutionary program that we offer is based on the clients' individual needs which we group them together like a classroom type setting where consumer participation is optional depending on their capabilities. We will encourage leisure-like type of an environment where everything will work as a role and play setting.

Part of the services we will provide is therapy and personalized counseling which shall includes:

a. Aromatherapy
b. Smell and touch interactive to stimulate tactile and olfactory kills and senses
c. Arts and crafts sessions
d. Physical exercises
e. Habilitation training
f. Mental exercises
g. Games and recreation activities
h. Singing "Karaoke" time
i. Musical instrument plays
j. Movie time
k Talent time
l. Habilitation training
m. Day Club or Sports Bar and Dance

15. SALES FORECAST

Based on our sales forecast, the months of January, February, March and April are our slow months in operation where we await the result of the program statement evaluation and approval coming from Community Care Licensing and Inland Regional Center. We expect to officially start receiving consumers by May and June 2004 when word has gone out to the public that there is a new unique day care center in town. By the month of May 2004, we expect to receive referrals of approximately five consumers for our community based program. By the succeeding months, we expect the referral to increase by as much as 15 to 25 consumers as we will start our center based operation with an expected consumer referral of at least 15. We assume sales growth by as much as 30% during our first three quarters of our operation and projected attainment of a full house capacity within less than 8 months from date of initial operation.

GRAPH: SALES MONTHLY

Table 3.0 Sales Forecast

16. MILESTONES

The accompanying table list important program milestones with their corresponding target dates and budget allocations. For the purposes of our milestone, during the months of September, October and November, we expect to have a final determination of our commitment and a clearer picture of our corporate path and challenges. Within the said months, our program design will be in progress and expect to submit our plan with the Community Care Licensing and Inland Regional Center for initial review and evaluation. We will expect a 90 day review of our program design which we expect to execute by the early months of 2004 preferably between January and March. During those slow months, we will be purchasing equipments, acquire site facility location and an office as well as staff hiring and training by January 2004. By the month of April 2004, our program design will be approved and ready for initial operation.

Table 16.0 Milestones

17. MANAGEMENT SUMMARY

Our initial management team shall compose of the following who receives mentoring from the Board of Directors:

    Board of Directors:
    Onlee Sample, President
    Onlee Wan, Vice President
    Sample, Secretary
    Sample, Treasurer

Regional Director for Programming/ Administrator : Onlee Sample

Program Director: Open

Assistant Program Director: Wan Sample

All of the members of our management team shall comprise of the Regional Director/ Administrator, Program Director, Assistant Program Director and health care consultants, therapist, behaviorist, psychologist, psychiatrist, LVN, RN, social worker and other team players are experienced in the health care field.

18. PERSONNEL PLAN

The initial set of personnel shall consist of Regional Program Director / Program Administrator, Assistant Program Director and the Program Director which shall hire initial number of direct care staff and support staff of 3 for the first month in operation. As the population of consumers increase, so is the number of staff to be increased in proportion to the consumers enrolled in the program. Our staffing ratio starts at a modest of 1:6 depending on the type of consumers. However, when the company starts accepting behavior consumers as well as those with considerable amount of community involvement and social recreation, the number of staff shall be increased considerable in proportion to the program statement as the needs of the clients being served.

Table 18.1 Personnel Plan

19. FINANCIAL PLAN

The plan is to initially operate the business in a cost effective form where the company shall locate a program site that is at least 2000 sq. ft at a rent cost of approximately $1.25 per sq. ft sufficient to accommodate an average of 60 consumers at a one time. However, bear in mind that the program shall consist of three different components namely: Center Based, Community Based and Leisure Center. During the first three months of operation, the center shall accept for its first stage in business consumers at a Community Based program. Then, after the site has been approved for official occupancy, the center shall accept Center Based consumers as well as consumers for its Leisure Center program by the fourth and fifth month of operation. The center shall take into serious consideration that it shall be accepting during its first month of operation community based clients to be able to generate funding sufficient for its initial operating costs. As the demand for our service grows, we will be expanding our site to encompass a neighboring office to be able to meet our growing needs.

The most important factor is the availability of the program site as soon as the vendorization requirements are met.

Part of our assumption is that the estimated start-up cost is limited to less than $45,000 to be able to meet our obligations for at least four to six months to cover our operating cost.

By our estimates, we expect to receive clients by the third and fourth month from the time we open our doors to business.

20. IMPORTANT ASSUMPTIONS

Our important assumptions are as follows:

1. That there is no delay in our projected operation timeline.

2. That we will be able locate a training facility that is situated strategically to cover our target areas.

3. That our program design will be accommodated accordingly by Community Care Licensing and Regional Center.

Table: 20.1 General Assumptions

21. BREAK EVEN ANALYSIS

Our break even projection is at $18,240 which we aim to accommodate at a minimum at least 12 consumers per day for at least 21 days per month to cover our basic operating cost. Our expected break even point shall occur during the first six to eight months of operation to recoup our cost. The estimated price per consumer served is at $ 65.00 per day at 21 days in a month. We assume that all the consumers will be able to participate actively on a daily basis to be able to benefit from our services.

Graph: 21.1 Break Even Analysis

Table: 21.1 Break Even Analysis

22. PROJECTED PROFIT AND LOSS

Our projected profit and loss (as indicated on our table) shows that during our first six months of operation, we expect to accommodate our first batch of five (5) consumers by the month of May and June after consistent marketing. On said months, we will be generating a gross sales of approximately $6,825.00 each month. During said months, we project a negative net profit/sales of approximately (-$12,797.00) but by July of same year, our projected revenue will be at $ 22, 475.00.00 which is equivalent to approximately 16 consumers being served. By the following year 2005, our company would be known to the neighboring cities and the success of our prototype is starting to become popular not only among residential care facilities, but also with Regional Center. Therefore, our projected revenue is at $1,661,400.00 by 2005 and by the year 2006, our income should have doubled at $2,130,600.00 which is at 96.38 % in Gross Margin.

Table 22.1 Profit and Loss Statement

23. PROJECTED CASH FLOW

For our cash flow projections, aside from the $26,899.00 start up funds we will use in purchasing equipment and supplies for our start up operations, we still have to infuse additional $ 18,240.00 to offset for our expected losses during the initial months of operation in January, February, March. By April 2004, we project a negative cash flow of approximately $12,797.00 which will require investors to once again infuse approximately $ 5,000.00 to even out shortage in cash flow. During the difficult months of May, June and July where we will be expecting shortage on revenue, we are looking at possibly an input of additional capital in the amount of $ 10,000.00 in order for our cash flow to retain a positive cash flow of approximately $ 37,265.00. We project that with the help of a progressive marketing as well as continued support from Inland Regional Center, we will maintain our positive cash flow position and that our projected income will gradually increase at a consistent phase of 25% growth to 35% on a monthly basis. With our introductory service catering for the community based activities, we will on a gradual phase introduce to the public our center based as well as our leisure center programming. Because of this new addition to the services we offer, we project income to grow with the demand as it arises.

Graph: 23.1: Cash Flow

24. PROJECTED BALANCE SHEET

Projected Balance Sheet indicates that our starting balance is $25,000.00 which by the following year 2005, our cash balance is $521,381.00 and by our third year of operation, our cash balance is at $1,299,628.00 In our first month in operation, we shall have at least $40,000.00 in net worth and by the end of the first year of operation, our net worth is $226,882 and by the third year of operation, it is estimated at $1,112,106.00 to $ 2 Million Dollars as net worth.

Table 24.1: Balance Sheet

USEFUL CONTACT INFORMATION

Associations
American Health Care Association
1201 L St, NW
Washington DC 20005
(202) 842-4444

American Society on Aging 833 Market St, Ste 511
San Francisco, CA 94103
(415) 974-9600 *www.asaging.org*

California Association for Health Services at Home
723 S St., Sacramento, CA 95814
(916) 443-8055
www.cahsah.org

California Association of Adult Day Services
921 11th St, Ste 701
Sacramento, CA 95814 (916) 552-7400
www.caads.org

California Association of Health Facilities
2201 K Street
Sacramento, CA 95816
(916) 441-6400 *www.cahf.org*

California Association of Homes and Services for the Aging , 7311 Greenhaven Dr, Ste 175 Sacramento, CA 95831   (916) 392-5111
www.aging.org

California Association of Residential Care Homes
2380 Warren Road, Walnut Creek, CA 94595
(925) 937-3046

California Center for Assisted Living
2201 K Street, Sacramento, CA 95816
(916) 441-6400, *www.ca-assistedliving.org*
National Center for Assisted Living
1201 L St, NW
Washington DC 20005

(800) 434-0222; (202) 842-4444 *www.ncal.org*

State Government
California Department of Aging
16 K Street
Sacramento, CA 95814
(916) 322-3887
- Office of State Ombudsman
(916) 323-6681
www.aging.state.ca.us

California Department of Health Services
P.O. Box 942732
Sacramento, CA 94234-7320
(916) 445-4171
www.dhs.ca.gov

California Department of Social Services
744 P Street
Sacramento, CA 95814
(916) 657-3661
www.dss.cahwnet.gov

California State Capitol
Governor's Office
(916) 445-2841 *www.governor.ca.gov*

State Government Information Line
(916) 322-9900 *www.ca.gov*

Federal Government
White House
(202) 456-1414 *www.whitehouse.gov*

Insurance Resources
California Partnership for Long Term Care
714 P Street, Room 616
Sacramento, CA 95814
(800) 434-0888
www.dhs.ca.gov/cpltc

Health Insurance Counseling and Advocacy Program
(800) 434-0222
www.aging.state.ca.us/html/programs/hicap.htm

Other Resources

Area Agencies on Aging (*www.cahf.org/public/consumer/areaagcy.php*)

The California Department of Aging contracts with a statewide network of 33 Area Agencies on Aging (AAAs) which are responsible for the planning and delivery of community services for older persons and persons with disabilities. (800) 510-2020

Eldercare Locator (*www.eldercare.gov/*)
A nationwide toll-free information and referral service
(800) 677-1116

Regional Centers for Persons With Developmental Disabilities (*www.cahf.org/public/consumer/ddregctr.php*) Regional centers are responsible for coordination of services and case management for persons with developmental disabilities, as well as diagnosis and assessment, preventative services to parents and persons at risk of having developmental disabilities, individual program planning, advocacy, monitoring and evaluation.

Statewide Ombudsman

(*www.cahf.org/public/consumer/calombud.php*)
Each county has a Long Term Care Ombudsman program, whose goal is to advocate for the rights of all residents of long-term care facilities and adult day health-care centers in the state.
(800) 231-4024

Glossary of words

ADMINISTRATOR: "Administrator" means the individual designated by the licensee to act in behalf of the licensee in the overall management of the facility. The licensee, if an individual, and the administrator may be one and the same person.

ADULT: "Adult" means a person who is eighteen (18) years of age or older.

AMBULATORY PERSON: "Ambulatory Person" means a person who is capable of demonstrating the mental competence and physical ability to leave a building without assistance of any other person or without the use of any mechanical aid in case of an emergency.

APPLICANT: "Applicant" means any individual, firm, partnership, association, corporation or county who has made application for license.

APPROPRIATELY SKILLED PROFESSIONAL: means an individual that has training and is licensed to perform the necessary medical procedures prescribed by a physician. This include but is not limited to the following: Registered Nurse (RN), Licensed Vocational Nurse (LVN), Physical Therapist (PT), Occupational Therapist (OT) and Respiratory Therapist (RT). These professionals may include, but are not limited to, those persons employed by a home health agency, the resident, or facilities and who are currently licensed in California.

Activities of Daily Living (ADLs): The physical functions necessary for independent living. These usually include bathing, dressing, using the toilet, eating and moving about (transferring).

Acute Hospital - A hospital which provides care for persons who have a crisis, intense or severe illness or condition which requires urgent restorative care.

Area Agencies on Aging (AAA): Local government agencies which grant or contract with public and private organizations to provide services for older persons within their area.

Assisted Living/Residential Care Facilities for the Elderly (RCFE) – Personal care and safe housing for people who require supervision for medication and assistance with daily living, but who do not require 24-hour nursing care.

BASIC RATE: "Basic Rate" means the SSI/SSP established rate, which does not include that amount allocated for the recipient's personal and incidental needs.

BASIC SERVICES: "Basic Services" means those services required to be provided by the facility in order to obtain and maintain a license and include, in such combinations as may meet need of the residents and be applicable to the type of facility to be operated, the following: safe and healthful living accommodations; personal assistance and care; observation and supervision; planned activities; food service; and arrangements for obtaining incidental medical and dental care.

CAPACITY: "Capacity" means that maximum number of persons authorized to be provided services at any one time in any licensed facility.

CARE AND SUPERVISION: "Care and Supervision" means those activities which if provided shall require the facility to be licensed. It involves assistance as needed with activities of daily living and the assumption of varying degrees of responsibility for the safety and well-being of residents. "Care and Supervision" shall include, but not be limited to, any one or more of the following activities provided by a person or facility to meet the needs of the residents: Assistance in dressing, grooming, bathing and other personal hygiene; Assistance with taking medication, as specified in section 87575; Central storing and distribution of medications, as specified in section 87575; Arrangement of and assistance with medical and dental care. This may include transportation, as specified in section 87575; Maintenance of house rules for the protection of residents; Supervision of residents schedules and activities; Maintenance and supervision of resident monies or property; Monitoring food intake or special diets.

Chronic: A lasting, lingering or prolonged illness.

Copayments: Copayments are those payments made by an individual at the time that he or she uses health care services. Copayments are generally a set amount depending upon the specific service received.

Custodial Care: Care is considered custodial when it is primarily for the purpose of meeting personal needs and could be provided by persons without professional skills or training.

COMMUNITY CARE FACILITY: "Community Care Facility" means any facility, place or building providing non-medical care and supervision, as defined in section 8701.c.(2).

CONSERVATOR: "Conservator" means a person appointed by the Superior Court pursuant to the provisions of section 1800 et seq. of the Probate Code to care for the person, or person and estate, of another.

CONSULTANT: "Consultant" means a person professionally qualified by training and experience to provide expert information on a particular subject.

CONTROL OF PROPERTY: "Control of Property" means the right to enter, occupy, and maintain the operation of the facility property within regulatory requirements. Evidence of control of property shall include, but is not limited to the following:

A Grant Deed showing ownership; or The Lease Agreement or Rental Agreement; or A court order or similar document which shows the authority to control the property pending outcome of probate proceeding or estate settlement.

DEFICIENCY: "Deficiency" means any failure to comply with any provision of the Residential Care Facilities Act for the Elderly and regulations adopted by the Department pursuant to the Act.

DEPARTMENT: "Department" is defined in Health and Safety Code, section 1569.2(b).

DIETICIAN: "Dietician" means a person who is eligible for registration by the American Dietetic Association.

DIRECTOR: "Director" is defined in Health and Safety Code, section 1569.2(c).

DOCUMENTATION: "Documentation" means written supportive information including but not limited to the Licensing Report (Form LIC # 809).

Developmental Disability (DD): Disability which originates before age 18; can be expected to continue indefinitely; constitutes a substantial handicap to the disabled ability to function normally; and is attributable to mental retardation, cerebral palsy, epilepsy, autism, or any other condition closely related to mental retardation which results in similar impairment of general intellectual functioning or adaptive behavior.

Durable Power of Attorney for Health Care: This legal document authorizes the person given the power to make decisions regarding the person's medical treatment only when the person giving the power becomes incompetent.

ELDERLY PERSON: "Elderly Person" means, for purposes of admission into a Residential Care Facility for the Elderly. A person who is sixty-two (62) years of age or older.

EMERGENCY APPROVAL TO OPERATE: "Emergency Approval to Operate" (EAO) means a temporary approval to operate a facility for no more than 60 days pending the issuance or denial of a license by the licensing agency.

EVALUATOR: "Evaluator" means any person who is duly authorized officer, employee or agent of the Department including any officer, employee or agent of a county or other public agency authorized by contract to license community care facilities.

EVIDENCE OF LICENSEE'S DEATH: " Evidence of Licensee's Death" shall include, but is not limited to, a copy of death certificate, obituary notice, certification of death from the decedent's mortuary, or a letter from the attending physician or coroner's office verifying the death of the licensee.

EXCEPTION: "Exception" means a variance to a specific regulation based on the unique needs or circumstances of a specific resident or staff person. Requests for exceptions are made to licensing agency by an applicant or licensee. They may be granted for a particular facility, resident or staff person, but cannot by transferred or applied to other individuals.

EXISTING FACILITY: "Existing Facility" means any facility operating under a valid unexpired license on the date of application for a new or renewal license.

GUARDIAN: " Guardian means a person appointed by the Superior Court Pursuant to the provisions of section 1500 et seq. of the Probate Code to care for the person, or person and estate, of another.

HEALING WOUNDS: include cuts, stage one and two dermal ulcers as diagnosed by a physician, and incisions that are being treated by an appropriate skilled professional with the affected area returning to its normal state. They may involve breaking or laceration of the skin and usually damage to the underlying tissues.

HOME ECONOMIST: "Home Economist" means a person who holds a baccalaureate or higher degree in home economics and who specialized in either food and nutrition or dietetics.

IMMEDIATE NEED: "Immediate Need" means a situation where prohibiting the operation of the facility would be detrimental to a resident's physical health, mental health, safety, or welfare. Examples of immediate need include but are not limited to:

A change in facility location when residents are in need of services from the operator at the new location; A change of facility ownership when residents are in need of services from the new operator.

INSTRUCTION: Means to furnish an individual with knowledge or to teach, give orders, or direction of a process or procedure.

Home Health Agency (HHA): A home health agency is a public or private agency that specializes in giving skilled nursing services, home health aides, and other therapeutic services, such as physical therapy, in the home.

Hospice: A hospice is a public agency or private organization that primarily provides pain relief, symptom management, and supportive services to terminally ill people and their families in the home.

Intermediate Care Facility (ICF): An ICF provides health related care and services to individuals who do not require the degree of care or treatment given in a hospital or skilled nursing facility, but who (because of their mental or physical condition) require care and services which is greater than custodial care and can only be provided in an institutional setting.

Institutes for Mental Disease (IMDs): Provide supplemental special programs for mentally disordered individuals in a locked and/or secured skilled nursing facility setting.

Long-Term Care Insurance: A policy designed to help alleviate some of the costs associated with long term care needs. Often, benefits are paid in the form of a fixed dollar amount (per day or per visit) for covered LTC expenses.

LICENSE: "License" is defined in Health and Safety Code section 1569.2(g).

LICENSEE: "Licensee" means the individual, firm, partnership, corporation, association or county having the authority and responsibility for the operation of a licensed facility.

LICENSING AGENCY: "Licensing Agency" means a state, county or other public agency authorized by the Department to assume specified licensing, approval or consultation responsibilities pursuant to section 1569.13 of the Health and Safety Code.

LIFE CARE CONTRACT: "Life Care Contract" is defined in Health and Safety Code, section 1771(m).

Managed Care: Medical care delivery system, such as HMO or PPO, where someone "manages" health care services a beneficiary receives; each plan has its own group of hospitals, doctors and other health care providers called a "network"; usually promote preventive health care; may have to pay a fixed monthly premium and a co-payment each time a service is used.

Medicaid (Medi-Cal in California): The state medical assistance program which provides essential medical care and services for individuals and families receiving public assistance, or whose income is not sufficient to meet their individual needs. Sixty-five percent of residents in skilled nursing facilities rely on Medicaid.

Medicare: The nation's largest health insurance program, Medicare covers 37 million Americans. Medicare provides insurance to people who are 65 years old; people who are disabled; and people with permanent kidney failure. Medicare provides only limited benefits for skilled care, and under specific guidelines, for nursing home and home health care. Only 8 percent of individuals in skilled nursing facilities rely on Medicare.

Medicare Supplementary Insurance: This insurance pays the 20% of the Medicare approved amount of which Medicare pays 80%.

Medigap Insurance: Medigap insurance are private insurance products that provide insurance protection for the costs of hospital services that are rendered to a Medicare beneficiary that exceed the amount Medicare will pay for the hospital services.

NEW FACILITY: "New Facility" means any facility applying for an initial license whether newly constructed or previously existing for some other purpose.

NON-AMBULATORY PERSON: "Non-Ambulatory Person" means a person who is unable to leave a building unassisted under emergency conditions. It includes, but is not limited to, those persons who depend upon mechanical aids such as crutches, walkers, and wheelchairs. It also includes persons who are unable, or likely to unable, to respond physically or mentally to an oral instruction relating to fire danger and, unassisted, take appropriate action relating to such danger.

NUTRITIONIST: "Nutritionist" means a person holding a master's degree in food and nutrition dietetics, or public health nutrition, or who is employed by a county health department in the latter capacity.

Occupational Therapy: Activities designed to improve the useful functioning of physically and/or mentally disabled persons.

Ombudsman: Individual designated by a state or a sub-state unit responsible for investigating and resolving complaints made by or for older people in long term care facilities. An ombudsman is also responsible for monitoring federal and state policies that relate to long term care facilities, for providing information to the public about the problems of older people in facilities, and for training volunteers to help in the ombudsmen program. The ombudsman program is authorized by Title III of the Older Americans Act.

Personal Care: Involves services rendered by a nurse's aide, dietician or other health professional. These services include assistance in walking, getting out of bed, bathing, toileting, dressing, eating and preparing special diets.

Physical Therapy: Services provided by specially trained and licensed physical therapists in order to relieve pain, restore maximum function, and prevent disability, injury or loss of a body part.

PHYSICIAN: "Physician" means a person licensed as a physician and surgeon by the California Board of Medical Examiners or by the California Board of Osteopathic Examiners.

PROVISION OR PROVIDE: Whenever any regulation specified that provision be made for or that there be provided any service, personnel or other requirement, it means that if the resident is not capable of doing so himself, the licensee shall do so directly or present evidence satisfactory to the licensing agency of the particular arrangement by which another provider in the community will do so.

PROVISIONAL LICENSE: "Provisional License" means a temporary, nonrenewable license, issued for a period not to exceed twelve months which is issued in accordance with the criteria specified in section 87231.

Respite: The in-home care of a chronically ill beneficiary intended to give the care-giver a rest. Can also be provided in a hospice or nursing home (as with hospice respite care)

RELATIVE: "Relative" means spouse, parent, stepparent, son, daughter, brother, sister, half-brother, half-sister, uncle, aunt, niece, nephew, first cousin or any such persons specified in this definition, even if the marriage has been terminated by death or dissolution.

RESIDENTIAL CARE FACILITY FOR THE ELDERLY: "Residential Care Facility for the Elderly" means a housing arrangement chosen voluntarily by the residents, or the resident's guardian, conservator, or other responsible person; where 75 percent of the residents are at least sixty-two years of age, or, if younger, have needs compatible with other residents as specified in section 87582; and where varying levels of care and supervision are provided, as agreed to at time of admission or as determined necessary at subsequent times of reappraisal.

RESPONSIBLE PERSON: "Responsible Person" means that individual or individuals, including a guardian, conservator, or relative, who assist the resident in placement assume varying degrees of responsibility for the resident's well-being. This includes the County Welfare Department, Adult Protective Services Unit, when no other responsible person can be found.

ROOM AND BOARD: "Room and Board" means a living arrangement where care and supervision is neither provided nor available.

SERIOUS DEFICIENCY: "Serious Deficiency" means any deficiency that presents and immediate or substantial threat to the physical health, mental health, or safety of the residents or clients of a community care facility.

Skilled Nursing Care: Care which can only be provided by or under the supervision or licensed nursing personnel. Skilled rehabilitation care must be provided or supervised by licensed therapy personnel. All care is under the general direction of a physician and necessary on a daily basis. Therapy that is needed only occasionally, such as twice a week, or where the skilled services that are needed do not require inpatient care, do not qualify as skilled level of care.

Skilled Nursing Facility (SNF): Provide 24-hour nursing care for chronically-ill or short-term rehabilitative residents of all ages.

Social Security: A national insurance program that provides income to workers when they retire or are disabled and to dependent survivors when a worker dies. Retirement payments are based on worker's earnings during employment.

Speech Therapy: The study, examination, and treatment of defects and diseases of the voice, speech, spoken and written language.

Sub-Acute Care Facilities: Specialized units often in a distinct part of a nursing facility. Provide intensive rehabilitation, complex wound care, and post-surgical recovery for persons of all ages who no longer need the level of care found in a hospital.

Supplemental Security Income (SSI): A federal program that pays monthly checks to people in need who are 65 years or older and to people in need at any age who are blind and disabled. Eligibility is based on income and assets.

SOCIAL WORKER: "Social Worker" means a person who has a graduate degree from an accredited school of social work or who has equivalent qualifications as determined by the Department.

SSI/SSP: SSI/SSP" means the Supplemental Security Income State Supplemental Program.

SUBSTANTIAL COMPLIANCE: "Substantial Compliance" means the absence of any deficiencies which would threaten the physical health, mental health, safety or welfare of the residents. Such deficiencies include, but are not limited to, those deficiencies referred to inn section 87451 and the presence of any uncorrected serious deficiencies for which civil penalties could be assessed.

SUPERVISION: means to oversee or direct the work of an individual or subordinate but does not necessarily require the immediate presence or the supervisor.

TRANSFER TRAUMA: "Transfer Trauma" means the consequences of the stress and emotional shock caused an abrupt, involuntary relocation of a resident from one facility to another.

VOLUNTARY: "Voluntary" means resulting from free will.

WAIVER: "Waiver" means a variance to specific regulation based on a facility-wide need or circumstance which is not typically tied to a specific resident or staff person. Requests for waivers are made to the licensing agency, in advance, by an applicant or licensee.

RESIDENTIAL CARE FACILITY'S COMMON TERMINOLOGY: ABBREVIATIONS

DSS - Department of Social Services
CCL - Community Care Licensing
CCF - Community Care Facility
ARF - Adult Residential Facility
CCLD – Community Care Licensing Division
CCF - California Code of Regulations
LPA - Licensing Program Analyst
COB - Central Operations Branch
OAL - Office of Administrative Law
ASP - appropriately skilled professional
SMP - skilled medical professional
EM - evaluator manual
DD - developmental disability
IPP - individual program plan
CDER- client development evaluation report
ARM - alternative residential model
SMA - schedule of maximum allowances
RVS - relative value scales
P & I – personal and incidental (records or money)

IHSS – in-home supportive services
CYA - cover your _ _ _!
COLA- cost of living adjustment
QUALITY ASSURANCE – Assuring services are of the highest quality
PROGRAM FLEXIBILITY – the allowance for and exception
APPRAISAL – an assessment or evaluation of a resident
RETENTION – maintaining, retaining, or keeping a resident
EXCEMPTION – requested for when employee has a criminal record
EXEPTION – requested for a specific resident or staff person in regards to a particular circumstance, or program
WAIVER – variance for a specific regulation not tied to an individual
COMPLIANCE – obeying and properly following the law

Made in the USA
Lexington, KY
18 November 2014